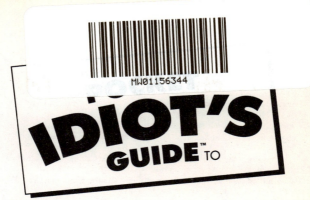

THE COMPLETE IDIOT'S GUIDE TO

Oral Sex

by Ava Cadell, Ph.D.

ALPHA

A member of Penguin Group (USA) Inc.

This book is dedicated to my husband, Peter Knecht,
"The Cunnilingus Guru."

Contents

Appendixes

Introduction

First I'd like to congratulate you for picking up *The Pocket Idiot's Guide to Oral Sex*. This book is for busy, adventurous people who want no-holds-barred, straight-to-the-point information on titillating, erotic, and luscious oral sex for men and women.

I have written this book so it will be fun and easy to find whatever question, technique, or fact you are looking for. It offers an expansion of your oral sex horizon with unique tips on sexercises for your genitals, advanced oral sex positions, how to achieve the ultimate orgasm, a TriGasm. It will help you to avoid oral pitfalls and even teach you the latest slang words for oral sex and your genitals.

Whether you are an oral sex virgin or an oral sex master, this book will be a valuable tool to ensure that you have the best oral sex experience possible, making every oral sex encounter a memorable one. I believe everyone can learn more about oral sex, and can become an outstanding lover. As a leading sex expert, I've been teaching thousands of singles and couples all around the globe how to have healthy sex and relationships for more than a decade. While writing this book, even I learned some new dynamics on oral sex.

Extras

To make this book more user-friendly, you'll come across fun sidebars containing extra bits of information that explain the topics and terms throughout the book. Use these as road signs for your oral sex tour to understanding and appreciating the art of oral sex. There are four types of sidebars:

Oral Info

These give you significant facts about oral sex, which can also be informative or cautionary.

Penis Talk

These are definitions concerning the penis or parts of the penis and how it works.

Sexploration

These are sex tips for making your oral experience better.

Vagina Talk

These are definitions concerning the vagina or parts of the vagina and how it works.

Acknowledgments

Thanks to Mikal E. Belicove, acquisitions editor at Alpha Books for Penguin Group (USA) Inc. for offering me the chance to write this book, and to Nancy Lewis, my editor, whose contributions were excellent and enjoyable. Special gratitude goes to my patient husband, Peter Knecht, who hardly saw me while I was working on this book; to Robbi Firestone, my right hand who managed to juggle running my company and analyzing my book simultaneously; to Kim Yaged, for her resourceful research; and to my stepson, Chance, who is now a master of slang.

Trademarks

Chapter 1

Attitudes About Oral Sex

In This Chapter

- Get familiar with slang oral sex terms
- Oral sex inhibitions
- Male and female sex myths
- Find out why men and women love oral sex

In this chapter, you'll get the down low on what exactly oral sex is, how to get rid of any sexual inhibitions you may have, and some of the benefits of oral sex. We'll examine why good girls were taught not to do it and why men are obsessed with it. We'll even answer the question, "Is there such a thing as bad oral sex?" This chapter will help you get rid of old notions and prepare you for a healthy oral sex experience.

What Is Oral Sex?

The medical term for oral sex is *irrumation*, which literally means "to suck." The technical term for oral sex performed on a man is *fellatio; cunnilingus* when performed on a woman. In our book, oral sex is the term used for all sexual activities involving the use of the mouth (lips, tongue, throat, or teeth) to sexually lick, kiss, suck, or nibble the male or female genitals. Orally satisfying the sexual organs should be pleasurable to both the giver and the receiver of oral sex. The male sexual organs, the female sexual organs, as well as the mouth and tongue are sensitive with lots of nerve endings.

Penis Talk

Oral sex on the genitals of a man is technically called **fellatio**, from Latin, *fellare*— "to suck." Fellatio is oral sex performed on a man's penis that may or may not be continued to orgasm and ejaculation.

Some people engage in oral sex instead of intercourse as a means of contraception (birth control), because pregnancy is not possible unless semen comes into contact with the *vagina*. Oral sex can be used for pleasure even when avoiding pregnancy is not a concern. Oral sex can be a prelude to sex, it can be the main event, or it can be a form of afterplay, too. The choice is yours and your partner's.

Oral sex can be enjoyed in a wide variety of situations:

- **As the receiver.** You can receive oral sex selfishly or as a loving gift. The more you trust your partner, the better oral sex will be. You'll have the confidence to play and have fun.

Vagina Talk

The **vagina** is the muscular passageway that leads from the uterus to the vulva. It is the birth canal, the passageway for menstrual flow to leave the body, and the area that receives the penis during sexual intercourse. Oral sex on a woman is technically called **cunnilingus,** which comes from the Latin words *cunnus* ("vulva") and *lingere* ("to lick").

- **As the giver.** Oral sex can be as pleasurable for the active person giving it as it can be for the passive person receiving it. I know one woman who claims to reach the best orgasms while she is giving her lover oral sex.
- **As the giver and receiver.** This is when one partner performs oral sex while the other receives it, but it can be performed by both partners at the same time in a *sixty-nine position,* named after the shape and form of the Arabic numeral 69.

What's in a Name?

I always thought it was ironic that so many terms for oral sex have become equated with negative situations or feelings. If a young man gets a parking ticket, he says, "That sucks!" Or if he fails to get the raise he wanted, he says, "That really blows!"

A common slang term for giving oral sex to either a man or woman is "giving head." Done on the genitals of a man, common slang is a "blow job," or BJ for short. Done on the genitals of a woman, common slang is "eating her out."

Most people usually use slang terms when talking about oral sex during sex. Another common euphemism, for both sexes, is the verb phrase to "go down on someone."

Oral Info

Although it is called giving a man a "blow" job, it is actually accomplished by sucking on the man's penis. The term *blow job* is believed to stem from eighteenth-century Europe, when prostitutes were called *blowers*. During the 1930s, prostitutes would offer to *blow off* their customers. It wasn't until the mid-1960s that the term *blowjob* was commonly used, after a film was released by Andy Warhol titled, *Blow Job*. In the film, there were several explicit descriptions of the act.

Slang Words for Cunnilingus

Over the years, giving oral sex to a woman has had many descriptive slang names ranging from gobbling, yummy it down, eating out, cunt lapping, polishing the pearl, plating, carpet munching, canyon yodeling, eating pussy, muff diving, frenching, alphabetizing, bag lunch, beaver dinner, bird licking, box lunch, fur-burger feast, bush doctor, cherry flip, chewing bubble gum, chow box, clam dinner, and the genital kiss.

Slang Words for Vagina

Many women are uncomfortable hearing or saying words like *twat, snatch, beaver, clam, slit,* or *cunt* because they think they have negative connotations. Most women are comfortable with the word *pussy* to describe their vagina, especially when it's used in a compliment like, "Your pussy looks beautiful." In contrast, the ancient *Tantric* (sacred and spiritual sex teachings) worship for women's genitals is illustrated by a host of lyrical words like *Jade Gate, Jade Chamber,* and *Golden Furrow.* The ancient Hindu term yoni has achieved some notoriety today and has more respectful overtones.

 Sexploration

As a verbal turn-on, it can be a good idea to say the slang words that you find the most erotic and then ask your lover to repeat them. If you tell your lover which words turn you on the most, you can both use them during love-making and oral sex.

Slang Words for Fellatio

Common slang terms for fellatio include blow job and sucking off. Also, to go down on, give head, 68 (you do me, and I'll owe you one), breathing through the ears, buff the helmet, buff the knob, butterfly flick, checking the mike, choking, chomping the chicken, cleaning your head, hum job, hummer, playing the skin flute, dick licking, and cock sucking.

Slang Words for Penis (and Testicles)

Men really don't have a problem with calling their penis by slang names. In fact, it turns most men on when a woman calls it a cock, especially if she says, "Your cock looks and feels so good." Other popular terms for the penis include arrow, baloney, woody, beaver cleaver, schlong, beef bayonet, pork sword, lap taffy, pecker, dick, prick, and bishop. Let's not forget about slang words for the testicles, which include balls, nuts, bag, cobblers, goolies, and the boys.

Name Those Genitals

Men and women also like to name their genitals or give each other's genitals pet names. Here are some popular penis names: Peter, John Thomas, Johnson, Godzilla, Mr. Happy, Long John, Tiger, and the Monster. Women like more sensitive or cute names for their vaginas like lotus, lily, petal, pearl, kitty, cookie, or coochie.

When couples name each other's genitals, they often use famous historical couples like Adam and Eve,

Caesar and Cleopatra, Napoleon and Josephine, or Bonnie and Clyde. I encourage this so couples can have fun talking about their genitals in public and others won't have a clue what they are talking about. For example, a guy might say something like, "How is Cleopatra feeling today?" She could reply, "Cleo would like to get some attention because she's feeling a little neglected." With that, he could answer back, "You tell Cleo that I've come to bury Caesar, not to praise him." It's all about communicating your wants and needs in a playful manner. I like to call sex *adult play* because too many people take sex far too seriously.

Oral Sex Begins with Self-Love

What do you think is the most common, universal sexual issue? No, it isn't penis or breast size, but the attitude looming behind your physical attributes that counts more than what you look like. And that manifests itself by causing us to feel inhibited. It is lack of self-worth, which leads to inhibition. Anyone who grew up on this planet has experienced this loss of self-esteem and self-value. It has many causes, from family conflicts to religious programming. What matters now is giving yourself a positive self-perception and permission to be yourself without guilt and shame. You've earned it. You deserve it.

Some people feel stress and are apprehensive about giving and receiving oral sex. It can feel intimidating having someone look at your genitals, and you may worry about what you smell like, taste like, or look like—it can be overwhelming. Sexual shame and guilt from past influences can create anxiety, but with self-love, you can overcome these negative feelings of insecurity.

Sexploration

I would like to encourage everyone to examine the inside and the outside of their sexual organs. Look at it in a mirror, get to know it, and learn to recognize any changes in your body. Just for fun, draw what you think your genitals look like.

Oral Inhibitions

Everyone is inhibited about something, whether it's physical appearance, performance as a lover, or the ability to let go and have an incredible orgasm. Some people are so inhibited about sex they have never explored their bodies. And if they don't know what arouses them, they surely cannot communicate it to a partner.

Statistics show that more than 80 percent of women have never explored the inside of their vagina and almost as many have never even looked at the outside. This is sad, because knowledge equals power! If you can't lovingly look at your own genitals, how can you be comfortable letting someone else experience them?

What Oral Sex Can Be

It's important to remember that oral sex at its best is a mutual giving and receiving. Here are some examples of what oral sex can be:

- Oral sex can be a precious gift to someone who is worthy to receive it. Our sexual gifts are as valuable as any other part of ourselves that we prize. Selecting the right sexual partner to give to and receive from is as important a decision as choosing anything you place a high value on.

- Oral sex can be a natural high, perhaps even the best of nature's uplifts. It can energize us and make us feel more creative afterward.

- Oral sex can be a wonderful form of self-expression, infinitely artistic. It is both beautiful and erotic. It is gentle and assertive. It is relaxing and energizing.

- Oral sex can be a way to renew stamina, not deplete it. It can free us from emotional stress and release any tension and discomfort lodged in our muscles.

But most of all, it is a unique connection between two people who want to share a divine pleasure.

What Oral Sex Shouldn't Be

It is equally important in defining oral sex to weed out what doesn't belong in its repertoire of images.

- First and foremost, oral sex is not a sin. It didn't make it to the top 10 commandments, so it must be okay! Besides, why would God have created a *clitoris* for a woman if it wasn't supposed to be stimulated? It has no other function than pleasure. (Read Chapter 2 for more information on the clitoris.)

Vagina Talk

The **clitoris** has absolutely no function other than orgasmic pleasure. It has the highest number of concentrated nerve fibers found in the human body—8,000 to be exact. That's higher than anywhere else in the body and twice as many as the man's penis.

- Oral sex is not dirty; it is not something to be ashamed of. And it is not unhealthy as long as proper protection is used. In fact, sexual fitness can improve your health, not take away from it.

- Oral sex is not perverted, because it is a natural human instinct and desire that is enjoyable for both the giver and the receiver.

- Oral sex is not love but is often confused with love. Sexual desire and love are similar in that the need to be close to somebody and the desire for fulfillment are related.

- Oral sex is not to be misused as a weapon. Withholding oral sex to punish a partner is a sign of poor communication and stored-up anger; it does not give power to the "withholder." To the other extreme, forcing one's self sexually on another person is a sign of inadequacy, not power or real strength.

- Oral sex is not a healthy addiction. A sexual addiction or compulsion is an escape from love.

- Oral sex is also not a sport; it is not merely a form of exercise. It is a full-body experience, not just mouth-to-vagina or mouth-to-penis.

To enjoy its many pleasures, oral sex is a journey, not just a destination.

Is Oral Sex Really Sex?

In the minds of many teenagers, oral sex isn't really sex. They seem to think they can stay virgins by engaging in oral sex because the girl's hymen isn't broken. That's like saying you can have anal sex and remain a virgin. Technically, it's true, but theoretically and emotionally it's not.

In my mind, it is ridiculous to view oral sex as "not sex." It's just as intimate as sexual intercourse, so why would you engage in oral sex with someone you wouldn't want to have intercourse with?

Some men even think they aren't cheating when they have oral sex with another woman because they can't get her pregnant. Believe me when I say that giving and receiving oral sex is considered one of the most intimate and erotic acts that can be exchanged within a loving adult relationship … and yes, it is sex!

Good Girls Don't Do That

During childhood and adolescence, women are often taught to fear sex. They are warned that good girls shouldn't lose their virginity; they shouldn't pleasure a man or themselves until after they are married. Here are some negative messages that can deeply affect a woman's attitudes toward sex:

- Don't touch yourself "down there," talk about sex, learn about sex, read about sex, get turned on, give in to sexual desire, be available, kiss on the first date, feel sexual, or be too forward.

- Do be attractive, be obedient, be passive, be sensitive, be nurturing, maintain a "good" reputation, wait for the man to initiate romance, and expect the man to know all about sex. Refuse a man when he asks you to be sexual, but also do whatever the man tells you to do after you're married to him.

These confusing sexual messages from society's projected attitudes can be quite damaging.

Bad Little Boys

Men can grow up thinking that sex is bad (even to the point of touching themselves) and that oral sex is dirty. They are typically influenced by strict parents, teachers, or religious intrusions who provoke feelings of guilt and shame. I had a client who wouldn't let his wife give him oral sex because she was the mother of his children. He was programmed to believe sex was only for procreation. I'm happy to report I helped change his attitude to a healthier outlook on sex. If you've been influenced by negativity toward your body or sex, I'm giving you permission to love your own body and your lover's. Sex counselors, therapists, and sexologists are qualified to help you overcome your sexual fears, so seek help if you need it.

Oral Info

Men as well as women have been trained to rigidly obey many cultural myths about themselves and their sexuality. If they don't live up to those myths, many of them suffer from guilt and negative feelings. For example, men worry unnecessarily about the size of their penis, when in fact the size of a man's heart is much more important to a woman.

Sexual Myths

Women and men are bombarded with sexual myths that have been passed down from centuries of sexual repression:

- You should only have sex with one person during your life.
- Your naked body is shameful and embarrassing.
- Sex is dirty and sinful.
- Sex is only for men's pleasure and for making babies.
- As a woman, if you have sexual desires, you are perceived as a slut.

- As a woman, never reveal you are sexually experienced, even if it's true.
- As a woman, fake your orgasm if you can't reach one.
- As a woman, your vagina should always be naturally lubricated.
- It is selfish and demanding to want clitoral stimulation.
- As a man, you must be able to get it up, keep it, and perform.
- As a man, hide your feelings of fear, inadequacy, or rejection.
- As a man, it's your job to give a woman her orgasm.
- As a man, don't be weak, be passive, or fail because you'll be a loser.
- It is selfish and demanding to want penile stimulation.
- You must have sex when your partner demands it, not when you want it.
- If you desire someone other than your partner, there is something wrong with you.

Can all these sweeping statements be true? If our genitals are as valuable as priceless rubies, why are they spoken of as "dirty"? If sex is so beautiful, why do people shame it? If sex is a no-no before marriage, how can we be expected to perform well and know everything about it on our wedding night?

It's no wonder women and men are often confused about sex; feel guilty, alone, and worried; are uncomfortable with their body; are waiting for *it* to happen; are in a hurry to get it over with; are masturbating in secret, if at all; and are worried about whether their genitals smell and taste normal.

Society's messages are obviously ignorant and have been handed down to us from times when people just didn't deal with "such matters." It's up to each individual to establish your own sexual values and overcome the taboos with self-knowledge, choosing options, being honest with yourself and others, knowing the facts, learning techniques, and sharing your needs with others. It's up to each man and woman to be responsible for their own pleasure.

Our Basic Sexual Rights

Our basic human rights extend to include our sexual rights, too. These include the following:

As adults, we have the right to engage in consensual sex.

We all have the right to a sex life, including people who are physically and mentally disadvantaged.

We are free to think of any sexual thought or fantasy.

We have the right to determine our own sexuality.

As adults, we are free to choose our own sexual entertainment in the legal marketplace.

We have the right to not be exposed to unwanted sexual behavior or materials.

For men and women to achieve a full and satisfying sex life, which is each individual's right, they need self-knowledge, facts, techniques, and honesty, all of which are available in this book.

Why Men Love Oral Sex

Men love getting oral sex from a woman because it's like having intercourse in her mouth. Her soft lips wrap around his penis and her wet tongue dances around it as her hot mouth sucks him deeper and deeper—this is the ultimate pleasure for many red-blooded men. I've never known a man to say, "I don't want oral sex, please stop." In fact, 90.5 percent say they love getting oral sex. It's a basic male instinct to seek oral gratification.

When a woman gives a man oral sex, he not only receives physical satisfaction, but he also gets the visual pleasure of watching his lover between his legs. A man feels like he's gone to seventh heaven when his lover orally worships his penis, especially if she's enjoying it. Even though this book is filled with endless oral sex tips and techniques, I must inform you that enthusiasm is still more important than talent.

Men love oral sex either because it gives him the feeling of being serviced by his lover, which results in a sense of power for him, or he gets gratification from being submissive to his lover while receiving oral sex. These men love to surrender their most precious body part to their lover so she can over-power him with her mouth.

Both the first and second emotions make a man feel accepted and valued by his lover, so there is an emotional and physical connection between them that takes them to a higher level of intimacy. It also makes a man feel confident and gives him high self-esteem, especially sexually.

Sexploration

When you are the receiver of oral sex, try expressing a sexual fantasy that includes you and your partner. Be as graphic as you can; and use words and phrases that turn you both on.

Why Women Love Oral Sex

Although it is more common to hear how men overwhelmingly love oral sex performed on them more than women do, many women out there love oral sex performed on them, too. If, as a woman, you have to ask why, then you have definitely bought the right book.

Some women claim to enjoy oral sex more than sexual intercourse. There is no risk of pregnancy, less chance of catching an STD, and it's the easiest way for many women to reach a climax. Emotionally, it allows a woman to surrender herself to the pleasure of receiving. Oral sex also helps make a woman feel sexually confident, uninhibited, and worthy.

Is There Such a Thing as Bad Oral Sex?

You bet there is. Oral sex can be bad if you have it with someone you don't like. If oral sex is forced, controlled, uncomfortable, or painful, it can leave lasting emotional scars. When the person you are

giving oral sex to is unclean or smelly, it's unforget-
tably bad. If oral sex is too quick or the environment
you are in makes you feel uncomfortable, it can be
bad. When you or your partner are in poor health
or stressed out, oral sex can be bad. Read how to set
the mood for oral sex in Chapter 4 and how to avoid
oral sex mistakes in Chapter 8.

The Least You Need to Know

- Oral sex can be just as satisfying for the
  giver as it can for the receiver.

- The more you trust your partner, the better
  oral sex will be. You'll have the confidence
  to play and have fun.

- Oral sex (and sexual intercourse, for that
  matter) is all about communicating your
  wants and needs in a playful manner.

- It's up to you to establish your own sexual
  values, overcome oral sex taboos, and be
  responsible your pleasure.

- To achieve a full and satisfying sex life, you
  need self-knowledge, facts, techniques, and
  honesty.

- Oral sex is just as intimate as sexual intercourse, so you shouldn't engage in oral sex
  with someone you wouldn't want to have
  intercourse with.

Chapter 2

Her Body

In This Chapter

- Understand her body
- Keeping the vagina in tip-top condition
- Avoid harmful female bacterial viruses
- Get the lowdown on STDs
- How women reach orgasm

In this chapter, you'll go on an anatomical journey and discover a woman's sexual organs. You'll empower yourself by learning the mystery of the female sexual arousal cycle. You'll understand why a woman's vagina shouldn't smell like flowers. And you'll get the facts on safer oral sex and have your safer sex supplies ready, before you need them. This chapter is one of the most serious in this book because it will improve your knowledge on female sexuality and teach you the medical risks of oral sex.

Her Body Parts

It's obvious that some people have bigger noses than others; not everyone has the same color eyes;

and lips can be small, large, thin, or full. The anatomic variety that makes each human face unique is also reflected all over our bodies, including our sexual organs. Like our faces, each vagina has all the essential parts, but they can differ in color, size, shape, and proportion. The fact is that the more you know about a woman's sexual anatomy, the better lover you will turn out to be. Don't expect every vagina to look the same, don't compare one vagina with another, and never critique one. Welcome and praise its originality and think of it as a snowflake—no two are identical. No matter what shape or size her vagina is, it will have no effect on her orgasmic ability.

Vulva

The vulva is the visible outer area of the female genitalia, including the pubic hair area (*mons veneris*). Some women never groom their pubic hair while others style and trim it, bikini-line wax it, or even shave it off completely because they like the way it looks and feels.

The vulva consists of various parts, and when it comes to oral sex, many of these parts are neglected. It's like sitting down to eat a freshly cooked artichoke and abandoning all the leaves to get to the center of the artichoke. It's true that the heart is the tastiest and most tender, but by slowly pulling the petals apart, sucking on each one delicately, you'll create more anticipation, get more nourishment, and still experience devouring the succulent heart of the artichoke.

Sexploration

Did you know that the less pubic hair you have, the fewer odors you'll have? Another advantage to having a slick vulva is that it's easier to lick, and the extra visual charge can really turn some guys on.

Outer Vaginal Lips

The first set of lips are the outer lips (*labia majora*), which are cushioned with fat and help protect the genitals inside, much like the male scrotum. The outer lips are naturally covered in hair and come in a variety of sizes, ranging from small to large, puffy to thin. The texture of the outer lips also differs from smooth to crinkled, and the color of the outer lips can range from pale pink to dark brown. The outer lips may be slightly apart, revealing the inner lips (*labia minora*), or they may hide the entire area. Having the outer lips of a woman's vagina licked and sucked can be extremely pleasurable for her.

Inner Vaginal Lips

The inner lips have no hair or fat filling. They stretch from one end of the vulva to the other, meeting at two corners. At one end they form a protective covering for the clitoris, and at the other end they meet at the *perineum*, the landing strip that separates the vagina from the anus. Rich in nerve endings, the inner lips can result in orgasm when lavished with oral sex because they are connected to the clitoris.

> **Penis Talk**
>
> The **perineum** is the area between the anus and the scrotum in men and the anus and vagina in women. Some people call it the *taint* because it taint butt or scrotum and it taint butt or vagina. I refer to it affectionately as a "landing strip."

Urethra

Unlike a man's penis, where the urethra serves for both urination and ejaculation, a woman has an opening to urinate from that's separate from the vagina. It's called the *urethra*, and it looks like a small bump. The urethra is located between the clitoris and the vaginal opening. Just like the man's urethral opening, it is very sensitive when stimulated and results in the urge to pee.

Hymen

The presence of a thin covering over the opening of the vagina is called the *hymen*. Medically, the hymen is thought to be a form of protection that prevents things from being inserted into the vagina.

Technically, it's supposed to indicate that the woman is still a virgin. However, the hymen can be broken when a woman inserts a tampon or engages in physical activity like bike riding or horseback riding. Physical sexual activity like fingering the vagina can also break the hymen. There's also evidence that sexually active women may still have intact, though stretched out, hymens.

Vaginal Opening

The vaginal opening is a hollow, muscle-lined tube that extends from its opening to the cervix, located deep inside the vagina. The vagina connects the woman's external and internal reproductive organs and can expand to many times its normal size, especially when the vagina becomes the birth canal through which the baby passes from the uterus to the vaginal opening. It's a real treat when a woman gets her vaginal opening licked and orally penetrated.

Clitoris

Many women find it easier to reach an orgasm while they are receiving oral sex than when they are having sexual intercourse. Most intercourse positions simply don't stimulate the clitoris as directly as a talented tongue can. This is an anatomical fact because the clitoris is located above the vagina, making it difficult for the penis to stimulate it during penetration. The majority of women are able to reach a mind-blowing orgasm by receiving oral sex directly on or around her clitoris.

The clitoris consists of four parts:

- The head (glans) is the only visible part of the clitoris.

- Below the clitoral head is the shaft, which extends from the head to beneath the hood.

- Sometimes the clitoris can be difficult to locate because it's covered by a protective fold of tissue called the *prepuce*, or clitoral hood. In some women, the clitoral hood has several folds, making it even harder to find.

- The clitoris is located at the top of the inner lips (*labia minora*), where the lips are joined together.

If you can imagine the vagina as an ice-cream sundae, the clitoris is the cherry on top. When stimulated, the clitoris can grow up to three times its normal size, much like the penis. So it's no surprise that the clitoris is regarded as the female equivalent of the penis and the clitoral hood is equal to the foreskin.

Below the shaft and invisible to the eye are two small wings called the *crura*. They are one of the four parts of the clitoris.

The clitoris was designed to open sexual doors for women, literally. The very word *clitoris* derives from the Greek word for key, as in the key to female sexuality. It opens up women to pleasure. And for a woman to revel in and thoroughly enjoy sex, her mind must be in the right place and not constantly fighting the negative messages and myths mentioned in Chapter 1. The clitoris has its own rhythm and will not be rushed. A woman must have a connection from her brain, and the fantasies it activates, to her clitoris, thereby taking responsibility for her own satisfaction. If her mind is in harmony with her clitoris, she is moving with her own sexual rhythm.

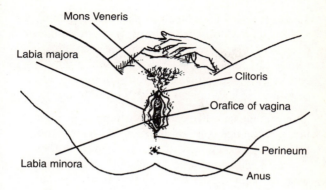

Female sexual organs.

The G-Spot

Because the G-Spot, or Goddess Spot as I prefer to call it, is not visible to the human eye, I'm not going to elaborate on it in this chapter. However, there are step-by-step instructions on how to find this mysterious spot and how to stimulate it in Chapter 10.

Keeping Her in Good Condition

First and foremost, a regular gynecological check-up (at least once or twice a year) for a pap smear is essential for all women. Your doctor can confirm the presence or absence of any medical problems like STDs (sexually transmitted diseases), cervical cancer, and proper healthy reproductive functions.

The best way for a woman to keep her vagina clean and healthy at home is to simply bathe it regularly with soap (preferably hypoallergenic soap) and water. The hood of the clitoris can sometimes collect the same gunk as the foreskin of the penis, so pull it back and clean it with a cotton swab.

The vagina is a self-cleaning organ and has a perfect pH balance containing friendly bacteria and lactic acid to keep it healthy and clean. It flushes out dead cells much like our nose dispels mucus when we blow it. To keep it hygienic, do not put anything unsanitary inside it. That includes dirty fingers, a penis that has penetrated the anus, unclean sex toys, foods, and oil-based products (just to name a few). My motto is, "If in doubt, leave it out." I will address this subject in more detail in Chapter 9. The bottom line is, when a woman's pH is out of balance, her natural secretions smell stronger and she is prone to getting infections.

The vagina is a normal exit for excretions, especially at the time of ovulation and menstruation. Under unhealthy conditions, the vagina will release excess mucous and waste from the body. If you are concerned with constant vaginal discharge, please seek a gynecological exam. He or she would be most qualified to assess the cause for the discharge and dispense the best treatment for it.

To Douche or Not To Douche

A healthy vagina does not need any douching. In fact, douching can change the pH balance of the vagina and cause infections. Many ingredients in douches are cosmetics and perfumes that can cause allergic reactions. However, when a woman is sexually active, it's more difficult for the vagina to maintain its clean and healthy status. Semen can introduce active bacteria and or viruses, which may combat the vagina's immune potential. That's why it's imperative for women to urinate right after sexual intercourse.

Yeast and Bladder Infections

One of the culprits that irritates the vagina and causes yeast infections is tight jeans, especially when worn without a barrier (no underwear). Wearing tight jeans can prompt the vagina to sweat and cause bacteria from the rectum to trickle into the vagina.

A nasty yeast infection (aginitis) can cause itching, discharge, and an unpleasant odor. Tips to prevent this from happening include wearing cotton under-wear and always wiping from front to back. The most common remedies for yeast infections are Monistat, an over-the-counter cream, and Diflucan, an oral prescription pill. Be aware that taking anti-biotics (like various forms of penicillin) can also create an overpopulation of yeast cells in the vagina, but eating yogurt can counterbalance the damage done by antibiotics.

Bladder infections, also known as cystitus and uri-nary tract infections (UTIs), can prompt constant urination and burning, so seek medical help as soon as you feel any abnormal symptoms. Your doc-tor will probably recommend Cipro XR by Bayer, which is designed to target the bacteria that cause UTIs. UTIs can be caused by having frequent sex with new partners, lack of lubrication during sexual intercourse, and bacteria from the rectal area.

The best way to avoid getting a UTI is to drink plenty of water; urinate after sexual intercourse; never hold urination in when you feel the urge to go; avoid using douches, spermicides, and intimate body sprays; wipe from front to back; and be sure the vagina is sufficiently lubricated before having sexual intercourse. Even using condoms that aren't adequately lubricated can cause too much friction and result in a UTI.

Oral Info

Some women swear that drinking cranberry juice helps relieve bladder infections. The cranberry juice produces more acidic urine, which in turn can help restore the natural balance of the urinary tract.

Lack of Arousal

Lack of arousal in women can be caused by a variety of things, including birth control pills, antidepressants, and hormonal changes. Fortunately, there is help for women to regain their sex drive. Initially, I recommend you go to your gynecologist and ask for a hormone test to determine if your estrogen or testosterone level is normal. If it's low, the doctor can give you a prescription for estrogen pills or injections. There is even an estrogen ring made of soft plastic that, when inserted into the vagina, emits estrogen on a gradual basis.

Testosterone patches and creams are available for those who need an extra boost of the sex hormone. Plus, there are lots of herbal supplements, aphrodisiacs, and topical ointments that claim to enhance arousal. If your hormone levels are normal, your lack of arrousal could be related to stress, fatigue, or lack of support from your partner. Psychological problems can result in low or no desire for sex, so if you're feeling out of sorts, seek help from a professional.

Taste and Smell Your Best

One of the most common reasons women don't enjoy receiving oral sex is because they fear their genitals will smell or taste bad. The truth is that a woman's flavor and aroma is influenced by her monthly cycle, diet, medications, vitamins, stress level, and even her environment. As you might expect, if you eat healthfully, drink plenty of water, and keep your stress level down to a minimum, you'll taste your best. The natural taste of a woman's vagina can span from slightly sweet, salty, tangy, to even a trace of iron around the time of her menstrual cycle.

Plenty of people find the natural body aromas much more arousing than the reek of pungent perfumes and intimate body sprays with names like "spring rain" and "autumn flowers." Our sense of smell is the strongest factor in sexual attraction. There's nothing dirty or unpleasant about genital odors and secretions (except in the case of certain vaginal infections, which can result in an unpleasant odor).

If you feel that a little body odor goes a long way, you might be more comfortable taking a shower or bath, or sponge-bathing each other before oral sex. When it comes to oral sex, cleanliness equals confidence.

Sexploration

I encourage everyone who hasn't already done so to try smelling and tasting their own sexual juices. To enjoy oral sex, you have to enjoy your own sex organs—this means appreciating everything about them.

Here's a healthy drink that will make you taste and feel great. However, I'm not sure any bartender will know of it by name: the vagina cocktail. Put the following three ingredients in equal parts in a glass with or without ice: orange juice (here's your vitamin C for overall good health), cranberry juice (helps prevent urinary infections), and pineapple juice (has the most healing components of any fruit). If you have a blender, add a tablespoon of your favorite yogurt (it can prevent yeast infections).

Better She Be Safe Than Sorry

If you love yourself, you must protect yourself. Ladies, there's no reason why you can't enjoy the eroticism of oral sex and practice safer sex at the same time. Even if you're in a monogamous relationship, you'll want to have some of the safer sex supplies around to help you add more pleasure, diversity, and spontaneity to your oral sex adventures.

Along with the information here on female codoms, dental dams, as well as latex gloves and finger cots, be sure you check out the, "Better He Be Safe Than Sorry," section in Chapter 3 on condoms and lubricants.

Female Condoms

Most female condoms work the same way. They're made of polyurethane (stronger than latex) and are hypoallergenic, heat conductive, and odorless. They are a soft, loose-fitting sheath specifically designed to protect women from pregnancy and STDs by lining the inside of her vagina.

Reality Condoms are the most well-known female condoms, but they recently changed their name to FC Female Condoms. Femidom is another brand of female condoms.

Read the instructions before inserting it because if you don't insert it correctly, it's like not using protection at all. The female condom has to go deep inside the vagina and over the cervix.

Dental Dams

Aptly named because they are used by dentists to isolate a tooth, dental dams come in various sizes and flavors. Made of ultra-thick latex, these square-shape barriers allow good sensations for oral sex. Sheer Glyde Dams are FDA (Food and Drug Administration) approved for protection against

STDs for cunnilingus and rimming. The best way to use a dam is for the giver to mark his "mouth" side of the dam so he knows which side he's going to lick, then apply a couple drops of lubricant on the other side, press the dam against her vagina with two hands, and enjoy.

Latex Gloves and Finger Cots

Good oral sex involves the hands as well as the mouth. There's nothing more exciting than orally pleasing a woman's clitoris and fingering her vagina or anus simultaneously. By using latex gloves and finger cots (think of them as mini-condoms for your fingers), you can increase erotic sensations and protect the receiver from jagged fingernails, cuts, germs, or viral STDs such as herpes, which can be spread by skin-to-skin contact.

STDs from Oral Sex

The list of STDs that follow describes the most contagious and common STDs when it comes to performing and receiving oral sex. Although no one knows exactly what the degree of risk is, to ensure safer sex be sure you have no cuts or lesions in your mouth or on your genitals. Protect yourself and your partner by using a barrier to avoid the contact of bodily fluids that may result in spreading a sexually transmitted disease.

Herpes is a virus that causes sporadic flare-ups of painful blisters, usually around the mouth and/or genitals. Herpes can hop from mouth to mouth and from mouth to genitals through the mucous membranes and skin. It can be spread by hand-to-vagina or hand-to-anus contact. Herpes is a common virus. You can get a prescription drug called Valtrex, and take one a day to prevent outbreaks of the virus.

Genital warts are similar to herpes in that they are a virus that remains in your system for life. They are spread in the same way, through skin-to-skin and mucous membrane contact. Warts can appear on or in the vagina and anus; they can even be found as far back as on the cervix. Treating genital warts is more extreme than treating herpes. The warts have to be removed surgically by laser, and the bad news is that they may reoccur anyway.

Gonorrhea is a serious bacterial STD that can be spread through unprotected oral-vaginal contact. Symptoms may not show, but vaginal burning, discharge, and pelvic pain are common warning signs. The good news is that antibiotics do work, but they must be taken for weeks to cure gonorrhea.

Syphilis is a severe bacterial STD that can also be spread through unprotected oral-vaginal contact, especially if there is a sore present on the mouth or vagina. Syphilis can be deadly if it isn't cured in the first couple stages. The first visible sign and stage is a sore at the entrance of the vagina; the second sign is a body rash. Fortunately, penicillin can cure syphilis in the early stages. However, the third stage attacks the nervous system and debilitates the heart. Medications have limited success if the disease is left untreated for too long.

Crabs and pubic lice are tiny creatures that gravitate toward the pubic hair, where they live. They can be spread from one infested person to another. It's possible to catch crabs and lice from a toilet seat, bedding, and even clothing. Symptoms include itching, swollen lymph glands, and a mild fever.

Hepatitis A is a dangerous virus that can be transmitted by rimming or analingus (licking or penetrating the anal opening with your tongue). Hepatitis A can be prevented by getting a hepatitis A shot. Symptoms may appear within one month after contact. In some cases, hepatitis infection can cause muscle ache, fever, loss of appetite, headaches, or dizziness.

> **Oral Info**
>
> Other rimming risks include anal herpes, anal warts, internal parasites, and even HIV.

Hepatitis B can be a life-threatening virus transmitted from sexual contact or contaminated needles. It's found in blood and other body fluids, such as semen, vaginal secretions, and breast milk. It's possible to contract hepatitis B when performing unprotected oral sex, especially when fluids from a carrier enter your body through a cut or sore in your mouth. Symptoms of hepatitis B are fever, abdominal pain, jaundice, and in some cases liver disease. There is no known cure, but it can be prevented with a vaccine.

Hepatitis C is the most deadly of all the hepatitis diseases. It is transmitted exclusively through direct blood contact, so the receiver of oral sex must be menstruating and the person going down on her must have a cut or sore on his mouth. There is no known cure or vaccine for hepatitis C at this time. Symptoms include the same as for A and B, plus dark urine, light stool colors, yellow eyes or skin, and tenderness of the liver area. There is no known cure, but it can be prevented with a vaccine.

HIV/AIDS can be fatal when the blood, semen, vaginal secretions, or breast milk of an infected person enters another person's bloodstream through a cut, sore, or blood vessel. If you perform oral sex on a menstruating partner, you could be at risk. If you have recently flossed or brushed your teeth, it's possible that you cut your gums and you could be at risk. HIV doesn't have any immediate warning signs, so it's possible to have the virus for years without knowing it—and to transmit it to others. The first symptoms of AIDS are weight loss, night sweats, pneumonia, and other illnesses related to a debilitated immune system. There is no known cure or vaccine for AIDS, but combinations of medications can slow down the virus.

Her Stages of Sexual Arousal

How does a woman know when she's had an orgasm? With an orgasm, the muscles of the pelvic floor always contract. If this doesn't happen, it may feel good, but it's not an orgasm.

A study of the sexual response cycle was first carried out by Masters and Johnson in the 1960s, when they studied more than 10,000 response cycles. They described the sexual response cycle as having four stages: excitement, plateau, orgasm, and resolution. I believe there are actually five cycles for a woman, with the first being foreplay.

Orgasm Cycle #1: Foreplay. Most women need to be prepared for sex with some foreplay. Whispering her name in her ear and then kissing her will release pleasure endorphins that will flood her brain with feel-good hormones like serotonin and dopamine. Blood flow will increase to her genitals, and her body will become sensitive all over. Now she's ready for the next stage of sexual arousal.

Orgasm Cycle #2: Excitement. Sexual excitement affects the entire body with the increase of her heart, pulse, and respiration rates. During this cycle, her breasts swell and her nipples become erect. Also, her vagina becomes wet and her clitoris grows up to three times its normal size.

Orgasm Cycle #3: Plateau. Her body temperature rises and changes the color of her inner vaginal lips to a deep red. Her clitoris retracts under the clitoral hood. Her uterus pulls upward into the abdomen, widening the vaginal space and allowing the penis to fit comfortably.

Orgasm Cycle #4: Orgasm. In the orgasm cycle, the uterus, anus, leg muscles, face, and hands begin to involuntarily contract. There are strong contractions in the vagina at 0.8 second intervals, 40 breaths per minute, and a heart rate that can go as high as 180 beats per minute.

Orgasm Cycle #5: Resolution. Cooling down is defined by how long it takes for a woman to get her pulse rate back down to normal and let the rush of blood to her pelvis subside. Blood pressure and pulse gradually return to pre-arousal levels. Swelling in the genitals and other areas decrease. The labia minora return to their normal color. Muscles relax, and organs and tissues resume their original positions.

Sexploration

During the resolution cycle, stay with your partner and hold her close. This physical connection after oral sex or any other kind of sex is most significant for a woman. It makes her feel like you care about her.

Orgasms vary between women and for the same woman at different times. There is no right or wrong kind of orgasm. Feelings will vary with kind and degree of stimulation, but also with how the woman feels about herself, her partner, and their relationship. Orgasms are described in many different ways but, in common, there is a sensation of building "pressure" or "tension" followed by a sense of inevitability once it starts and "relief" or "release" when it's finished.

The Least You Need to Know

- Every vagina is slightly different in the way it looks, but they all work the same.

- A regular gynecological check-up and pap smear are essential for women to maintain good health.

- Because the vagina is self-cleaning, douching is unnecessary and can upset the vagina's natural pH balance.

- You can acquire an STD from giving or receiving oral sex, so practice safer sex at all times.

- The female orgasm is a five-part journey, not just a destination.

Chapter 3

His Body

In This Chapter

- Get to know the penis
- Nip penis problems
- Condom fashion shows
- Dealing with STDs
- Discover his orgasm cycle

In this chapter, you'll get to know the penis and all its parts from the head to the anus. There'll be no more worries about the taste of semen after you read this sweet recipe. Whether it's a case of jock itch, impotence, or prostate enlargement, this chapter has the lowdown on the symptoms and treatments for whatever ails you. You'll also find out what condoms are best for oral sex and how to tell if your lover has an STD.

His Body Parts

All men are concerned about the size and appearance of their penis, and every guy knows exactly how long his erection is. The average length of an erect penis in the United States is 5.1 inches, but most guys dream of sporting a longer and thicker yardstick.

If you're wondering how that size compares to the rest of the world, consider that America is a melting pot of many nations and races, so in our country, we run the gamut of small, medium, and large, with the average size of 5.1 inches.

The most sensitive part of a woman is her clitoris and the first two inches inside her vagina, so if a penis is two inches or more, there's no reason why it can't satisfy a woman sexually.

Penises come in a variety of sizes, shapes, and colors. From long and skinny ones, short and chubby ones, curved ones, hairy or hairless ones, all penises have redeeming qualities. No matter what the penis looks like, a man should learn to love and accept it just the way it is, and a woman should learn to worship it. Always remember, it's what you can do with it that counts.

The Penis

The penis is a man's sexual and reproductive organ. The penis is made up of two parts, the *shaft* and the *glans*. The main part of the penis, the shaft, contains the tube (*urethra*) that drains the bladder. The urethral opening is located on top of the glans where urine and ejaculate (containing *sperm*) come from.

The Urethra

The urethra stretches from the bladder to the penile opening—where urine and semen exit, but not at the same time.

The Glans

The glans is the head of the penis and, whether circumcised or not, is exposed when a penis is fully erect. This area has the largest concentration of nerve endings in the penis, and men enjoy extra oral stimulation around the glans. The word *glans* comes from the Latin word for "acorn."

Foreskin

All boys are born with a foreskin or a covering over the tip of the penis. If a penis is uncircumcised, this layer of skin will cover the glans when the penis is soft (*flaccid*). Once it's erect, the foreskin will draw back to expose the glans. The foreskin is equivalent to the clitoral hood. Inside the foreskin is a layer of thin skin similar to the inner labia in women. Link-ing the foreskin to the penis is the frenulum, which is where the foreskin is removed during a circumcision.

Penis Talk

The most sensitive area on a man's penis is commonly known as his "sweet spot," clinically referred to as the **frenulum** and located underneath the head of the penis. This area calls for extra oral stimulation.

Frenulum

The frenulum is located just below the glans on the underside of the penis, where the circumcision scar appears. If uncircumcised, the frenulum is in the same location, below the tip of his penis, where the inner skin of the foreskin's hood meets the outer skin of the penis. The frenulum is a hotbed of sensitive nerve endings.

The Scrotum

The scrotum is located below the penis. Joined at the base of the penis, this puckered sac hangs and houses the testicles. Most men do not have perfectly symmetrically hanging balls. Usually one hangs a little lower than the other. The scrotum protects them from injury much like a helmet protects a motorcyclist's or a football player's head. The scrotum also works as a temperature control device. When it's cold, the muscles in the scrotum will contract, lifting the testicles protectively closer to his body. When the temperature heats up, it relaxes and lets them hang down. For the production of healthy sperm, the testicles need to be around 5 degrees below body temperature.

When a man gets fully aroused, just before ejaculation, the muscles in the scrotum will contract and his balls will rise, pulling them closer to the base of his penis. This is the point of no return.

Perineum

The perineum is the stretch of skin between the anus and the scrotum. Just below the skin of the perineum is where the root of the penis lies, and when he gets an erection, the perineum feels hard, too. The perineum is often a neglected erogenous zone just waiting to be stroked and licked.

Testicles

Also known as the *testes*, the testicles lie inside the scrotal sac behind the base of the penis. These globes of pleasure produce the sex hormone testosterone, and sperm are also generated here. Inside the testes are lots of tubes that produce the sperm, called *seminiferous* tubes. They open into the *epididymis*, where sperm is gathered and put in storage for six weeks. When it's ready, the sperm travels through the vas deferens up to the urethra. Regular ejaculation is healthy because the old sperm can be released, leaving room for new sperm to be replenished.

Most men love having their testicles orally lavished, but their biggest complaint is that some women are too rough.

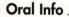

Oral Info

Did you know that the testicles are about 4 or 5 degrees cooler than the rest of a man's body temperature, providing the perfect conditions for sperm production? Avoid sitting in hot tubs and wearing tight briefs if you're trying to conceive.

Anus

The anus, the opening at the end of the digestive tract joining the rectum, is only few inches long. It's surrounded by the anal sphincter muscles.

Rectum

The rectum is 5 to 7 inches longer than the anus and is located at the lower end of the large intestine, leading to the anus.

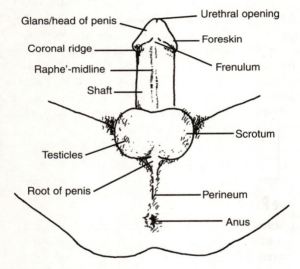

Glans/head of penis

Coronal ridge

Raphe'-midline

Shaft

Testicles

Root of penis

Urethral opening

Foreskin

Frenulum

Scrotum

Perineum

Anus

Male sexual organs.

Penis Parts You Can't See

Because many of the internal parts of the penis can be felt by stimulating it externally, let's review some of the most significant parts:

- The penis contains two chambers inside the shaft, *corpus cavernosum* and *corpus spongiosum*, which are spongy erectile tissue that fill up with blood and harden the shaft and head of the penis during arousal. There is no bone in the penis.

- There are two vas deferens tubes passing sperm from each testicle to the urethra. Your partner can feel the vas deferens (the tubes that from the testes to the prostate) with her fingertips if she applies pressure to the per-ineum, between the scrotum and the anus.

Oral Info

Vasectomy is a surgical procedure where a small segment of the tube is cut so sperm can no longer get through. The end result is sterilization.

The Prostate

Located beneath the bladder, the prostate gland is a walnut-shape organ that produces the prime ingredient in semen. It's accessible through the anus about 2 to 3 inches inside toward the front of his body. The prostate is also considered to be the male version of the G-spot. When stimulated, the prostate can provide orgasmic pleasure for some men, especially when it's combined with fellatio. There's more on the prostate and sexual arousal in Chapter 11.

As men age, the prostate may have a propensity to enlarge and could partially block the flow of urine, so regular prostate examinations are mandatory. We'll talk more about how to keep a prostate healthy later in this chapter in the "Prostate Problems" section.

Keeping Him in Good Condition

Obviously, if you want your genitals to taste and smell their best, you should bathe just before your oral sex encounter. For uncircumcised men, it's important to pull back the foreskin and clean underneath it where dead skin can build up and create an unpleasant odor.

Even when you take care of your pride and joy with the utmost attention, unexpected penis problems can raise their ugly head. Here are a few prevalent problems with solutions.

Jock Itch

Jock itch is common in athletes and people who are overweight or sweat a lot. It's a fungal infection of the skin that can be caused by not drying yourself properly after you bathe. Symptoms include itching in the groin and anal areas. A reddish rash will appear and may spread down the inner thighs. Blisters can also appear around the penis and scrotum areas, but not directly on them.

The best treatment is good hygiene and skin care. Over-the-counter topical antifungal gels and powders are also available. Tolnaftate and undecylenate are well-known, effective medications. The powder form is also useful as a drying agent. Clotrimazole (Fungoid, Lotrimin, Mycelex) and Miconazole

(Micatin, Monistat Derm) are also available over-the-counter and are effective against all fungi. Because it's contagious, don't share your clothes and have your own towels and wash them often so you don't pass jock itch on to others.

Impotence

Experts say that impotence affects between 10 and 15 million American men, and it implies that a man is unable to sustain an erection sufficient for orgasm. Impotence can be a total inability to achieve an erection or a tendency to have only brief erections. But it's not necessarily a permanent problem.

Erections can be affected by physical factors, such as high blood pressure or diabetes, as well cholesterol-filled arteries blocking the blood flow to the penis.

Some emotional factors responsible for impotence include stress, depression, anger, sadness, fear, or performance anxiety. They can all make an erection go away—or never happen.

Oral Info

It may be that you have a psychological block about a situation with your partner, who isn't turning you on as much as she used to. Communicate with her and ask her to stimulate you the way you like it. Try to relax, and your erection might come back on its own if there's no pressure.

Although there are many oral drugs, like Viagra, Levitra, and Cialis to treat impotence, there are also alternative techniques where a drug such as prostaglandin-E (a vasodilator) is actually injected into the penis and forces a rush of blood into the penis, thereby creating an erection.

The good news is that impotence is treatable in all age groups, and awareness of this fact has been growing. To help determine the cause, you should discuss the problem with a medical doctor familiar with your health history.

Oral Info

Medical studies confirm that smokers are twice as likely to become impotent because smoking damages the blood vessels in the penis, inhibiting the healthy flow of blood that leads to an erection.

Peyronie's Disease

The most common symptoms of Peyronie's disease are a curvature in the shaft, a lumpy or hard area in the penis, and painful erections. It's possible to injure the penis during very vigorous sexual intercourse. Forceful twisting or bending can also tear the tissue of the penis. Or the injury may be a result of a medical procedure like catheterization in which a tube is put into the bladder to pass urine, or a cystoscopy, when the doctor looks into the bladder after a prostatectomy (removal of the prostate gland).

Because Peyronie's disease may heal without any intrusion, surgery is not recommended for one or two years after the signs and symptoms of the disease.

Treatment includes taking vitamin E and a B complex substance (para-aminobenzoate), steroid treatment, and chemical agents like verapamil (a calcium channel-blocker) and collagenase (an enzyme that breaks down connective tissue).

The hard deformed tissue can be surgically removed, but is only recommended in severe cases.

Testicular Health

You should inspect your testicles regularly for signs of lumps or swelling, an enlargement of one of them, pain, or a sudden collection of fluid in the scrotum. Even aches or discomfort in the lower abdomen can be signs of testicular cancer, so do not hesitate to see a medical professional if you have any of the symptoms in this chapter.

Prostate Problems

Signs and symptoms that the prostate needs medical attention range from difficulty urinating, feeling the need to urinate frequently, urgency to urinate, not being able to empty the bladder, and of course, pain or discomfort.

Once the cause of your prostate problems is evaluated, your doctor can decide how you should proceed. Two types of medication control the symptoms of an enlarged prostate: Alpha blockers and finasteride (Proscar, Propecia). Alpha blockers are medications used to block the effects of raised blood pressure and are effective in about 75 percent of men. For more information on prostate health, go to www.prostatehealthdirectory.com.

There are several surgical procedures for prostate cancer and other severe prostate maladies, including transurethral resection of the prostate, transurethral incision of the prostate, or the open prostatectomy.

You Are What You Eat

If you intend to ejaculate in your lover's mouth—with her permission—you should be sure your sperm tastes as good as it can. In Chapter 2, on her body, I recommended that women taste their own sexual juices before receiving oral sex from their lover. I'm going to make the same suggestion to the guys. If you want a woman to taste you, then you should be prepared to taste yourself, too.

Lots of things affect the flavor of a man's semen, such as stress and other maladies. When you don't feel well, your body is not going to taste healthy. Also, smokers taste more bitter than nonsmokers; avid coffee drinkers, garlic and asparagus eaters, and even meat eaters tend to taste more acidic than others. To keep your semen smelling and tasting better, drink lots of water and eat lots of fruit, especially pineapple and melons.

Better He Be Safe Than Sorry

Many people are unclear on the risks associated with oral sex. Unprotected oral sex carries a lesser risk for

the transmission of STDs than unprotected intercourse or anal penetration, but there's still a risk
for both the giver and the receiver of oral sex. First
let's look at how to avoid these contagious STDs by
practicing safer sex.

Condom Talk

For party guys, condoms come in eight different
colors plus a brand that glows in the dark. Various
scents and flavors are also available for oral sex. Life-
Styles flavored condoms are actually just scented;
Durex both colors and scents its condoms, while Trustex appears to have the largest variety of scented and
flavored condoms. When enjoying sex with scented
condoms, the aroma permeates the entire room.

Today's condoms are high-tech wonders, featuring
anatomically sophisticated shapes, innovative designs,
and space age materials. Visit www.condomania.com
to purchase the most pleasurable condoms and lubricants on the market today. Here's the condom revolution: You can now buy custom-fit condoms, too.
There are 55 sizes to ensure that every guy, from 3
inches to 10 inches, can get a condom that fits properly for maximum security, comfort, and pleasure.

Store your condoms in a cool, dark place. Exposure
to sunlight, heat, or humidity can break down latex,
causing it to rupture or tear more easily.

Unopened condoms are usable up to four years after
the date of manufacture. Always check the date. Some
dates are marked "MFG," which is the manufacturing
date. Others are marked "EXP," which is the expira-
tion date, after which the condom should not be used.

Do not use any lambskin or natural condoms because they are not effective in the prevention of STDs. If a condom breaks, try to figure out why the condom broke so you can prevent it from happening again. Remember that safe sex begins with you!

Lubricants

We all know "wetter is better." I highly recommend you use some lubricant with all kinds of safer sex supplies. But which lube, oil, or potion is best for your individual needs? It can be very confusing because there are so many to choose from. I suggest an odorless, tasteless, water-soluble lubricant with a lighter consistency and without Nonoxynol-9 spermicide. Here are some of my favorites: Wet Light, Astroglide, ForePlay Personal Gel, Aqua Lube, Sensua Organics, and Probe Silky Light.

 Sexploration

Good Head Gel by Doc Johnson Enterprises is one of my favorite oral sex enhancements. It's for people who want to add some pizzazz to the flavor of their partner's genitals. It's available in mint, cinnamon, cherry, strawberry, and passion fruit flavors. It's worth buying for the "The History of Fellatio" article that comes inside the 4-ounce box.

Visual Cues for STDs

There are many types of STDs and, therefore, a wide and varying range of symptoms. Although many STDs have visible symptoms, many do not. Others, like syphilis, exhibit symptoms that disappear when the disease gets worse.

Any rash or discharge from the penis or her vagina should be checked by a physician—especially if it's painful or smells bad. Open sores around the anus, mouth, or genitals are an obvious warning for caution.

Condoms and safer sex techniques are always appropriate when having sex with anyone other than a long-term, strictly monogamous partner. As a relationship develops, before agreement to sexual activities, you should not be afraid to ask some basic questions. It's not easy—but it's imperative. You want to find out not only her overall attitude to sex, but also those sex practices relevant to your health.

In this day and age, anything other than a straight-forward approach emphasizing your concerns would be less than prudent. Explain that you are interested in having sex with her, but that you need to feel comfortable with the kind of sex you plan to have.

You should also read the information in Chapter 2 on STDs you can get from oral sex. They include herpes; gonorrhea; syphilis; crabs; hepatitis A, B, and C; and HIV/AIDS. Be sure to educate yourself by learning how to avoid these viruses and how to protect you and your lover against all STDs.

The most important thing to remember when practicing safe sex is to avoid the exchange of bodily fluids. If you are not in a monogamous relationship and you choose to have oral, vaginal, or anal sex, always use a barrier.

His Stages of Sexual Arousal

It's good to know that when a man gets aroused, his erection begins with some kind of sensory and mental stimulation. Then impulses from the brain trigger the muscles of the erectile tissue in the penis, allowing blood to flow and create a hard-on. In Chapter 2, I outlined the female sexual response cycle, but men's bodies respond differently, and the more you know about how both sexes respond, the more you'll be able to enhance your sexual experience for you and your lover. Here are the four stages of a man's sexual arousal leading to his orgasm:

Orgasm Cycle #1: Excitement. Whether his sexual excitement is created by physical or mental stimulation, the result is the same. His blood flow is increased to his genitals, and the penis, perineum, and prostate begin to harden. His heart, pulse, and respiration rate raise, too.

Orgasm Cycle #2: Plateau. The head of his penis becomes engorged with blood and swells. For the uncircumcised man, the penis head pushes out of the hole in the foreskin. At the urethral opening, some men secrete more pre-ejaculatory fluid than others, which is commonly known as "pre-come." This fluid contains semen, so practice all the necessary safer sex precautions to protect yourself and your lover from STDs and pregnancy.

Orgasm Cycle #3: Orgasm. His blood pressure rises and muscle tension builds to a peak as he's about to reach his orgasm. The testicles rise up close to his penis while his prostate gland is filled with fluid, ready to burst. When his involuntary pelvic muscular contractions begin, there's no going back and the sperm shoots out of the urethral opening of his penis.

Orgasm Cycle #4: Resolution. This is when the body goes back to its normal pre-arousal state. Muscles relax, the penis becomes soft, and the testicles descend back to their usual place. Heart beat and breathing slows down, and lots of men feel so relaxed that they just want to go to sleep.

It's normal for men to feel sexually depleted after their orgasm. They need time (between 10 to 20 minutes) to regenerate their energy and their sperm. Some food and a beverage will help refuel the body. My suggestion is to have your snack ready and close by so you don't have to abandon your lover for a trip to the refrigerator.

Sexploration

The resolution cycle is different for a woman because she can continue to have more orgasms if vaginal or clitoral stimulation continues, whereas a man needs to rest.

The Least You Need to Know

- The frenulum, located just below the glans (head) on the underside of the penis, is the most sensitive and sensual area.

- If you want your semen to taste good, eat lots of fruit just before oral sex.

- If you suffer from any form of impotence, the good news is that it is treatable.

- Condoms can be fun to use for oral sex, especially when a woman puts a flavored one on with her mouth.

- You can't always tell if your partner has an STD simply by looking, so practice safer sex even with oral sex.

Chapter 4

Getting Ready to Go Down

In This Chapter

- Understand the importance of setting the mood
- Learn how to psyche yourself up for oral sex
- Find out what to say before you go down
- Get a lesson in putting a condom on with your mouth
- Telling it like it is

In this chapter, you'll learn everything you need to know before you go down. I'll start with how to create the right mood—there's more to it than soft lighting and sexy music. I bet you didn't know that if you psyche yourself up for oral sex, it will greatly impact your sexual experience. It's all in this chapter.

Communication is the number-one ingredient for a consistently successful sex life. Find out what to say before you have oral sex, how to ensure your mate uses a condom, and even how to convince your partner to sign a sex contract. Now, if getting naked in front of your lover is uncomfortable for you, don't fret, because you'll also learn a fun new way to disrobe each other.

Setting the Mood for Oral Sex 101

Just like setting the mood to watch the Super Bowl game, anything you do to improve the setting will make it better and more memorable. For the Super Bowl, you might want to have a well-situated big-screen TV, some comfortable seats with pillows for your back, the temperature not too hot or too cold, lots of fast foods, and plenty to drink. Now let's use the same analogy for setting the mood for oral sex. The perfect setting can turn any night into a romantic evening your lover won't forget. A few small changes can transform your home into a love nest.

The first requirement is cleanliness. You don't want to have oral sex on stained sheets, a messy sofa, or a dirty floor. Imagine your fantasy sex god or goddess is coming to stay with you and you want to impress him or her. Whether Britney Spears, Pamela Anderson, Beyoncé, Ashton Kutcher, Denzel Washington, or Mel Gibson is your fantasy guest, don't neglect your window coverings, because the eyes always go to the windows. Curtains or blinds should be dust free and spotless. Add a romantic ambience by dimming the lights and lighting candles. There are no limitations to the number of candles you can have, but be sure, if they are scented, not to overwhelm. Fresh-cut flowers make a place look welcoming. Find out what your lover's favorite flowers are before

you buy them. Soft pillows are an inviting addition
to lounge on. You can throw them on the bed, sofa,
even on the floor. Invest in a good stereo or sur-
round sound unit, but keep the speakers away from
the headboard. Ask your lover what kind of music
gets him or her in the mood and then buy it. Anything by Barry White, Sade, Andrea Bocelli, or
Luther Vandros is a good bet. You'll get additional
brownie points for adding an extra sensual dynamic
to your setting!

Sexploration

One of the things a person remembers the
most about the mood while they were receiving oral sex is the kind of music that was
playing.

Most of us care about where we're going to perform or receive oral sex, so you must have easy
access at any angle to the furniture you plan to
use. The bed is always a favorite, but I'm a great
believer in variety, so don't hesitate to christen the
sofa or coffee table (as long as it's sturdy) and enjoy
the floor with the comfort of your throw pillows.

Finally, your place is ready. It looks great, but
what's still missing? How about some fresh fruit
and tasty morsels to nibble on? Even if you go
out for dinner first, you might get hungry after
oral sex. Don't forget to leave out something
to wet your whistle—one of oral sex's necessities.

Your safer sex supplies should be close at hand in a box, a drawer, or a basket filled with condoms, dental dams, latex gloves, finger cots, and lubricants. A decorative box of tissues, baby wipes, or a clean hand towel at arm's reach completes your mood-setting 101 education.

Getting Psyched Up to Go Down

Psyching yourself up for anything prepares you mentally and emotionally, sometimes even physically. Whatever the challenge, is, you will be more capable of dealing with it. For example, before running a marathon, you would want to increase your physical endurance through cardiovascular exercise, increase your strength with weight training, watch what you eat, get plenty of sleep, and visualize yourself winning the marathon. You have to expect to win, because if you prepare for success but expect failure, you will get what you expect.

The fact that you've picked up this book on oral sex means you've taken the right step in preparing yourself for going down. You have the desire to learn everything you can to be a good lover, and you've taken action to make it happen. Give yourself a pat on the back. Even with the help of all the tips and techniques this book has to offer, you still have to do one thing: conceive it. Believe it, and you will achieve it!

In the sections that follow, the reluctant, novice, amateur, and experienced individual will each be briefly described along with how they can overcome their fear of going down.

The Reluctant

In sex, it has been said that those who have the courage to communicate and experiment will find the greatest gratification. If you are reluctant to give or receive oral sex, ask yourself why before rejecting it completely. If your reluctance stems from sexual shame or guilt, these negative attitudes can be changed into positive ones as long as you have the desire to change them.

If you genuinely don't like oral sex, then read no farther, because I don't believe anyone should do anything they don't want to. If, however, you have had some prior unpleasant experiences sexually, don't punish yourself or your new lover by being reluctant to enjoy oral pleasure with someone who's right for you. Disregard negative statements about the genitals being unclean, or advice of peers who have cautioned you that oral sex is taboo or sinful. Even though it's hard to shake these views as an adult, you have the ability to reprogram yourself. Start by admitting that your peers didn't know any better and realize that they probably said those things because that's what they were taught.

Create a relaxing atmosphere for yourself before you begin your voyage into oral sex. Meditate, relax in a bubble bath, get a therapeutic message, take a long walk, listen to music, or do whatever it takes to get yourself prepared for your sexual journey.

The Novice

As a novice, you may have little or no experience at oral sex, but you are receptive, not reluctant. It's important for you to chose the right partner, someone who is patient and worthy of your oral sex affections. Get to know this person as well as you can before you indulge in oral sex. To psyche yourself up, imagine you are watching a big screen of your oral sex adventures. Visualize what your partner is doing to you and what you are doing to him or her. Your partner is responding positively to everything you do. Both of you are having a great time. Use all your senses to feel the experience of giving and receiving oral sex; touch your body lovingly, smell your lover's natural scent, look at his or her body erotically, taste your lover's genitals, and hear your lover groaning with pleasure. Now you have discovered that the mind is the most erotic organ we have!

The Amateur

This is someone who has already experimented and had good, mediocre, or not-so-good encounters. Whatever you experienced in the past, ask yourself what you learned. If it wasn't great, ask yourself what would have made it better. Every person is unique, so don't make the mistake of comparing your past partners with your present one, especially out loud. Don't assume your new lover will be aroused in exactly the same way as your past lover, or even that you will have the same sexual experience as you had before. If you did something that drove your last lover wild in bed, there's no guarantee that it will have the same effect on your new lover. Enjoy the newness of your lover by exploring all his or her erogenous zones with your tongue. Don't be shy to let your lover know that you want to give the best oral sex he or she has ever had.

The Experienced

The experienced person obviously enjoys the art of oral sex and doesn't need to prepare themselves psychologically in the same way as the other three categories do. However, it's important to maintain curiosity whether you're with your lover for the first time or the hundredth time.

Always ask questions like, "What's your favorite oral sex position?" and don't be afraid to ask for constructive criticism and feedback. As an experienced oral lover, you must be sure you don't become too predictable, so maintain enthusiasm and be willing to try new things. Even if your partner isn't responsive to giving you feedback, be sure you communicate your needs openly and honestly. Chances are your partner will catch on.

What to Say in the Beginning

My motto is "Don't have sex until you've talked about sex." So how do you bring up the subject of oral sex? You can't just blurt out, "I want to get some head," unless you never want to see that date again. Some people consider oral sex more intimate than intercourse, while others view it just as foreplay. It's up to you to find out how your partner feels about giving and getting oral sex. The best way to start an intimate discussion like this is to talk about your thoughts on the subject. If you think oral sex is a prelude to intercourse, you can say, "One of the sexiest things about making love for me is giving and getting oral sex before we make love. What do you think?" This is an open-ended question, so your lover has to give you a substantial answer. Whatever his or her answer, be sure you acknowledge it and don't be judgmental.

For example, your lover (a guy) may respond by saying, "When I'm getting oral sex, I often get carried away and reach an orgasm before I want to." He may be feeling inadequate as a lover and blaming himself for having *premature ejaculation*. You can help him by letting him know that it's okay. Say, "We'll go slowly and you can tap me on the shoulder when you think you're going to come and then I'll get on top of you, rub my clit against your shaft, so we can climax together at the same time." He'll be reassured that you're getting your needs met and that he's okay just the way he is. If your response had been unkind or insensitive, it could make his premature ejaculation even worse.

Penis Talk

Premature ejaculation is when a man is not in control over the timing of his ejaculation and believes that it occurs too soon.

A woman might say, "Getting oral sex is the only sure way I know how to climax," in which case the guy can reply, "That's great. I'll go down on you first, and then you can do me." Another sure way to help build a woman's confidence is to say something like, "You look so delicious, I can hardly wait to taste you."

The Sex Contract

I've come up with a sexual consent form so lovers can talk about the sexual activities they want to engage in before they jump each other's bones. I also created this sex contract so there would be no confusion or miscommunication as far as sexual consent is concerned. This form is actually a way for a person to ask for permission to have sex with another person.

So you're probably wondering, "When should I whip out this sex contract and present it to my prospective lover?" It should be well before you take out the condom. The best time to discuss the sex contract is over dinner or after you've watched a movie and before you get into bed. You can broach the subject by asking your partner what they think about prenuptial agreements and other consensual forms, such as the ones you have to sign before your doctor will operate on you. You can also take it out, lay it on the table, and ask, "What do you think of this? Let's have some fun with this tonight by talking about what we want to do sexually." Of course you can write your own sex contract or you can download mine from either one of my websites at www.avacadell.com or www.sexpert.com.

It's not for everyone, but it can certainly open up a good conversation about sex.

Sexual Consent and Privacy Agreement

I, (name) _____, hereby declare under penalty of perjury that I am over 18 years old. I further declare that this agreement is of my own free will and that neither I nor anyone near or dear to me has been threatened with harm or embarrassment.

Both parties agree that this is a private agreement not to be disclosed to third parties except in case of accusation of sexual misconduct by (name) _____ of (state) _____. If he/she shows or makes public this agreement without accusation of sexual misconduct, it is agreed that he/she will be liable for damages for invasion of privacy, whether or not his/her signature appears herein.

By initialing _____, agrees to engage in all or some of the following consensual acts. Initial the following:

Kissing _____

Sexual fondling _____

Sexual intercourse _____

Oral copulation (mutual) _____

Unilateral copulation by _____ only

Other, to be specified: _____

I further declare that I am at this time not under the influence of alcohol, drugs, or medication and agree to engage in consensual sex with _____ and intend not to change my mind before the sex act is over. However, it is further understood that if I, for any reason, say the words "Code Red," that my partner agrees to stop instantly.

Signed: _____   Date: _____

Signed: _____   Date: _____

Condom Talk

I've heard so many excuses from guys who don't want to wear a condom, with little or no regard for their own safety or the safety of their partners against STDs. Here are some of the most common: "It's unromantic," "They fall off," and my favorite, "If she really likes me, she won't make me use one." So ladies, if you're not in a monogamous relationship, here are some answers you can use when a guy gives you a hard time:

Him: "I don't think condoms are romantic."
Her: "Just let me show you how romantic condoms can be."

Him: "You don't trust me, do you?"
Her: "It's not a matter of trust; it's a matter of health."

Him: "I don't like to use condoms."
Her: "I don't like to have sex without them."

Him: "I haven't had sex in years so I know I'm clean."
Her: "Thanks for being so honest, but let's use one anyway."

Him: "I can't feel anything when I wear a condom."
Her: "Let me provide you with some extra stimulation."

Him: "I'll lose my erection by the time I get it on."
Her: "Here, let me put it on for you with my mouth." (See the section that follows.)

Him: "I'm only going to skip a condom this once."
Her: "Once is all it takes."

Him: "Sorry, I don't have one."
Her: "That's okay. I do."

Him: "How come you have condoms on you? Did you plan to have sex with me?"
Her: "I made sure I had some because I really care about you."

Him: "Forget it. I'm not going to use a condom."
Her: "Fine. Then let's not have sex until we can work out our differences."

How to Put on a Condom with Your Mouth

Now that we've talked our partner into wearing a condom, even for oral sex, let's give the guys a treat by putting it on their penis with our mouths.

First it's a good idea to get some flavored condoms. Trustex appears to have the largest variety of scented and flavored condoms. Pick your favorite flavor from banana, strawberry, orange, vanilla, cherry, or spearmint.

Next, follow these steps:

1. Get your man's penis erect.
2. Put a drop of lubricant on the head of his penis.
3. Carefully remove the condom from the package.
4. Turn the condom inside out and place it inside your mouth with the tip of your tongue inside the receptacle end. Leave some room at the end for the semen.

5. Be sure the condom is inverted in your mouth so it will go on correctly when placed on the man's penis.

6. Push the condom onto the head of his penis using your lips, not your teeth.

7. Wrap your lips around the head of his penis and use a little suction on the end of the receptacle of the condom to insure enough room for semen.

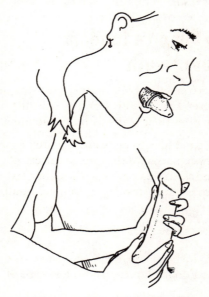

Putting on a condom with your mouth.

You may want to practice putting a condom on a cucumber, banana, or plastic dildo before you attempt it on your man's penis. Practice makes perfect, so have fun making safer sex enjoyable for both of you.

Aural Sex Will Enhance Oral Sex

Now that you've introduced oral sex into your sexual repertoire, it's time to heat up the conversation. Aural sex is to the ears what a mirror is to the eyes. It's intimate and erotic talk! Telling your lover what you like or dislike, or asking him or her what stimulation they enjoy can be nerve-racking if you haven't done it before. However, this is the perfect opportunity to direct your lover to pleasure you exactly the way you want. Remember, he or she can't read your mind.

How many of you will ask your partner how they would like their steak cooked? Now how many of you will ask how they would like their oral sex? You feel confident making dinner because you have taken the simple precaution of finding out how they like it. Isn't your relationship and sex life more valuable than a meal? Of course it is! You wouldn't consider ruining dinner for lack of asking your lover questions, so why risk the demise of a good relationship due to lack of communication when it comes to lovemaking? Feel confident that your communication skills reflect your lovemaking.

There's nothing wrong with telling your lover how you like or dislike to receive oral sex. If you don't like to have your testicles licked or sucked, say so up front, then she won't go there. If the only way you can reach an orgasm is by having your clitoris softly licked, then admit it before he gets started.

Everyone wants to hear sexy words of encouragement when they are being sexual. Ask yourself what you would like to hear your lover say to you when you're receiving oral sex. Most men like to hear graphic detail focusing on physical attributes like how big his penis is and how good it looks while women prefer to hear more emotional compliments like how sensual she feels and how good she tastes. Compliments are the bedrock of romance, so be generous with them, especially during intimacy. Most people feel vulnerable when their sexual organs are exposed, so letting him or her know that their sexual organs look great is a big plus. A woman can say, "I've been fantasizing about sucking you and feeling you hard and throbbing in my mouth." This will turn on any man. Tell your lover that he or she looks even better than your fantasy.

The best feedback you can give your lover is to show him or her how aroused you are by moaning and groaning with pleasure. Communication takes the guessing out of sexual performance. No more poking in the dark, at least not in silence. Sex talk can be used to turn a potentially bland meal into the tastiest and most tantalizing dish.

The Least You Need to Know

- Oral sex begins with your imagination, so psych yourself up for an oral adventure. Conceive it, believe it, and you will achieve it.

- To ensure your oral sex needs are met, talk about your oral sex preferences before you do it.

- Be open to healthy communication about oral sex and condoms so there is no confusion with sexual consent and safety.

- Erotic talk can enhance oral sex by adding sexual fantasy. You can make your fantasies come true by sharing them during oral sex.

Basic Techniques for Her

In This Chapter

- Orally loving his penis
- Why wetter is better
- How to use your hands
- Giving sex signals
- Get him to go down on you

In this chapter, you'll learn how to orally love your way around your man's penis. You'll understand why wetter is better and how sucking can be a learned subject that every woman can apply herself to, as long as she has the desire. You'll see how hand signals can communicate your oral needs and what to do to fake him out when he wants to come in your mouth.

A Beginner's Guide to Orally Loving His Penis

A recent sex survey claimed that 75 percent of men will only date a woman who gives oral sex. The good news is that any woman can learn to give great oral sex. All she needs is the desire and a good teacher. If you're reading this book, you have both.

The first thing you need to know about men is that they don't want you to take the long way around and they don't want to play teasing games. Men are goal oriented, and they want to know that they are going to get some head. Just like teaching someone to swim for the first time, the best tactic is often to throw them in the deep end. I'm going to suggest you do the same thing with oral sex; otherwise you may get too timid and come up with any number of reasons to back out.

He should lie on his back while you lie on your stomach between his legs. Get comfortable, because you could be in this position for a while.

Of course I don't expect you to put anything in your mouth without looking at it first, so take his penis in your hand and hold it with confidence, just like you would a gear shift on a car. Don't be afraid of it. His penis is a man's pride and joy, and it's your job to validate that by loving it when it's hard or soft, by kissing it, stroking it, licking it, and sucking it to keep it happy. As you inspect it, be sure there are no abrasions on it and that he looks clean and smells good. If his hygiene isn't up to par, suggest taking a shower or bath together. If he already looks appetizing, give him a verbal compliment right away. You can say, "You look so good. I can hardly wait to go down on you." Every man wants to hear that.

If you are not in a monogamous relationship, you need to practice safe sex and use an FDA-approved condom, even for oral sex. Read Chapters 2 and 3 for safer sex practices and plenty of condom talk. If you are in a committed relationship, have both been tested for STDs including HIV, trust each other implicitly, and have agreed to have unprotected sex, that's another story. In that case, your lover is probably comfortable with letting you see his penis when it's not aroused, and you should not wait until he has an erection before taking him into your mouth. While his penis is still flaccid (soft), wrap your lips around it and take it into your mouth so you can get used to it before it grows to its full potential. Here are some instructions on how to give your lover an oral treat.

Suck Him with Certainty

You may remember from Chapter 3 that the penis is made up of two parts, the shaft and the glans (head). Start by making sure you have plenty of saliva in your mouth (a dry blow job is as bad as no blow job).

Cover your teeth by wrapping your lips around them, then push your mouth down on your lover's penis, sucking (in slow motion) with your lips tightly closed (like sucking hard on a thick milk-shake to get the drink through the straw). Guys like to feel the sensation of a wet, warm, tight mouth sucking the penis. To impress him, open your mouth wide, relax your throat and move your mouth as far down over his penis shaft as you can. Even if this is only for a few strokes, it will let him know you are willing to try deep-throating. Don't use your hands yet. You've got to be able to give oral sex with and without hands. Hands can come into play, and we'll get into that later on in this chapter.

Right now, you have just lavished your man's penis with long, deep, sucking motions. While his penis is in your mouth, don't forget to breathe or you'll find yourself losing consciousness. Inhale through your nose every time you suck his penis into your mouth and then exhale through your nose as you lift your chin and release the penis. Also don't forget to swallow your own saliva frequently because it creates a distinct tugging sensation on his penis and adds more pressure around it. If his penis makes you feel like you are choking or gagging, move his penis to the side of your mouth into the hollow of your cheeks. Some men are flattered when a woman gags on their penis because it makes him feel like he is well endowed. Do not spit his penis out of your mouth, just move it to the side and take some deep breaths.

The Urethral Opening

If you want to change positions, ask him to hang his legs over the side of the bed, and you kneel between them with a pillow under your knees for comfort. This time, focus on the urethral opening, located on top of the glans.

Run the tip of your tongue over it from side to side like a windshield wiper. It's a very sensitive area, so don't overdo it, and don't try to wiggle your tongue

inside the urethral opening because that's not sexy.
Do maintain sexy confident eye contact with your
lover while you are licking him to let him know
you are enjoying yourself.

The Glans

Also known as the head of the penis, the glans is
one of the most sensitive areas and is equivalent to
the clitoris, with many concentrated nerve endings.

Hold his penis at the base with your dominant
hand and circle your tongue all the way around the
glans, clockwise then counterclockwise. Think of
the glans as a scoop of your favorite ice cream on
top of a cone. You don't want to miss a drop of that
tasty ice cream, so you greedily taste the top, lap up
the sides, and lick all around the cone, which is the
crown of his yummy penis.

The Frenulum

This is the most sensitive spot on the penis, so pay
special attention to its location. Look on the
underside of the glans where the inner skin of the
foreskin's hood meets in a heart shape. This is also
where the circumcision scar appears (if uncircumcised, the frenulum is in the same place). Begin by
licking his frenulum from side to side with quick,
darting flicks of your tongue. Then make an "O"
with your lips around the frenulum and use your
mouth to create some light suction on that area.
Imagine you are sucking a clam out of its shell.
Feel free to making sucking noises, because men
love sexy sound effects.

The Raphe

This is the penis seam, and it runs all the way from the head of the penis to the scrotum. It's even easy to find in the dark because you can feel the ridge of the seam with your fingers and your tongue. Here's an opportunity for you to lick the penis just like you would a lollipop, with long slurps. Start at the base of his penis, stick your tongue out as far as possible, and lick your way to the top of his penis.

The Scrotum and Testicles

The scrotum is the sac that hangs just below the penis and houses the testicles. They are part of his sexual package, so don't ignore them. Get familiar with them by caressing and gently massaging his balls of pleasure.

 Sexploration

Handle his testicles as if they are a precious artifact made of china. You want to admire them and hold them, but you don't want to damage them.

He can stand while you kneel in front of him or you can lie down on your back while he straddles you. The latter position is particularly good for access to his balls. You can kiss, lick, and suck on the scrotum by pulling it away from the testes, which are inside the sac. Imagine you are sucking on your lover's bottom lip with your mouth and imitate that same technique on his scrotum. *Absolutely no teeth allowed.*

This can be highly erotic for him, and he may request this oral method over and over again. It's easy to do because there's no gagging effect, and to make it even more erotic for him, ask him to masturbate while you suck on his scrotum.

The testicles are delicate like fresh farm eggs, so approach them cautiously yet sensually. Begin licking one ball at a time with the flat of your tongue in circular motions all around the testicle, letting your head follow suit (this is also a good neck exercise). Then give the other testicle equal attention until they are both sopping wet from your saliva. Next open your mouth wide and cup your lips gently around one of his balls while using the tip of your tongue to lick it in a circular action. Do the same to the other one and give them equal time. For the icing on the cake, use one of your hands to carefully push his testicles together and try to place them both in your mouth. There are more testicle-sucking techniques in Chapter 11.

The Perineum

Commonly referred to as the "taint" because it "taint balls and it taint butt," the perineum is the stretch of skin between the anus and the scrotum.

The perineum is located behind his penis, so it may be easier for you to access from behind. It is totally erotic for him. Ask him to lie on his stomach with his legs spread apart, then slide in between his legs and run your tongue along his perineum. Start by using the top flat part of your tongue in long broad strokes to lick him from the anus to the scrotum and then use the lower flat part of your tongue to lick from the scrotum to the anus. Next, with the point of your tongue, trace zigzags across his perineum as if you were a professional skier on a mountain.

Oral Combinations

What can feel better for a man than getting a blow job? How about getting a hand job at the same time? Stimulating more than one area simultaneously will automatically make you an oral sex specialist.

Sexploration

Some women admit that they are lazy when performing oral sex and can't be bothered to learn new techniques when the old ones work fine. If you think your guy is happy with a basic BJ and no frills, consider that some day he might be tempted by someone with a more extensive oral repertoire. If you're the best, then he's not going to wander.

Strum His Violin

Slide your prominent hand beneath his testicles, cup them together, and gently caress them with your fingers (be careful with your nails). Then take his penis in the other hand, and hold it firmly while you flick your pointed tongue back and forth over his frenulum. Imagine you are a musician strumming a violin with your tongue to make beautiful music. Your man's moans and groans will confirm that you are playing it correctly.

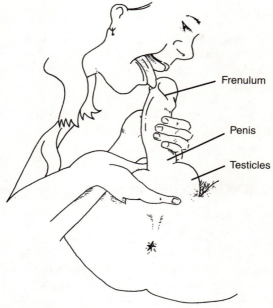

Strum his violin.

Vacuum and Brush

The best position for this technique is the 69 position with you on top. Make a tight seal around the head of his penis with your mouth and create a vacuum as you draw your head back, releasing his penis. While you continue to vacuum suck your man's penis, brush your fingernails lightly against his perineum as if you were a cat clawing your way up a tree. Scratch and brush both sides of your fingernails lightly from one end of his sexual landing strip to the other.

Bead It

Wrap a string of beads or pearls around his scrotum, tugging gently while sucking the glans. After a few minutes, let the beads dangle around his balls while you insert your index finger into your mouth and circle the head of his penis with it while you continue to suck on it. This stimulation makes a man feel like he's getting a blow job from two different women.

Why Wetter Is Better

If you want to enjoy giving oral sex, then you have to get used to the fact that it's going to be wet and sometimes sticky or messy.

A man's penis does not have as much natural lubrication as a woman's vagina. Even with the pre-ejaculation fluid, it's not enough to masturbate him with. The sexiest lubricant is your saliva, but don't just spit all over his penis. Drink some water if you feel dehydrated, fill your mouth with plenty of saliva, then let it drip over and down his penis as you take him into your mouth. You can rub it in with your hands if you are planning to masturbate him. No man wants a dry hand job. Or you can continue to give him oral sex, maintaining the wetness of his penis and balls. A man loves the feeling of warm, sloppy juices all over his penis. Drink some hot liquid prior to giving him oral sex so you don't "run dry" and lack enough lubrication to give him maximum enjoyment. He'll love the hot, steamy feeling around his penis. You can also gargle with mouthwash or suck on a mint prior to going down on him for a tingly fresh feeling you'll both enjoy. If things are getting too hot, suck on crushed ice while you give him oral sex. It will keep you from dry getting mouth and give him a frosty thrill.

How to Be Handy

One of the best things about using your hands is that you can use them as an extension of your mouth. They're especially handy if you don't want to or can't deep throat him. There's no doubt you will want to use your hands to steady his penis while you worship it orally. Hand contact also enables you to sensually caress other parts of his body such as his nipples and testicles while you're down there. You shouldn't be afraid to play with a man's testicles, but treat them like exquisite Christmas tree ornaments that can be broken with rough handling. Your hands can guide his penis in any direction you want and keep it from going too deep. Your hands can even mimic your mouth's actions if your jawbone gets too tired. But you'll need to use plenty of lubricant so he feels the warm moisture around his penis.

If you want to give your guy a great hand job, ask him to masturbate so you can watch how he likes it. Most women start by stroking a man's penis up and then down, but men prefer a smoother, rapid motion without stopping between strokes. The phrase "jerking off" is confusing because men don't really like a jerking motion at all! Don't be shy to ask him to show you what turns him on. He'll be impressed that you care and want to learn. Put your hand over his hand when he's masturbating, and try to duplicate his grip and the amount of pressure he uses.

Sexploration

A quick exercise to relax and get your jaw back into shape is to thrust your jaw forward, then down, then back, then to original position. You may want to go to the bathroom and do these while you empty your bladder or freshen up. It's quick, easy, and will get you back into the oral swing of things.

Another tip to remember is that when he ejaculates, don't stop masturbating him immediately unless he asks you to. Most guys appreciate a few extra strokes as they are reaching their climax.

I hope all this serious talk on how to use your hands hasn't given you sweaty palms, because there is a playful side to using your hands, too. Let your fingers dance around his genitals as you run them around his testicles and up and down his shaft. Wet your fingers with your saliva, then stroke the outside of his anus and tickle his perineum. Pump him up by squeezing his penis in the palm of your hand. And last but not least, give him a hand job with a twisting motion from the base to the tip, as if you were twisting half of an orange on a juicer. Guys tell me that this method of stimulation is the cat's meow.

Sex Signals

Signals can be very useful, particularly when your mouth is full and you can't talk. Agree on various sex signals before you get down or before you do something you're uncomfortable with. He can let you know that he's about to climax by patting you on the shoulder twice so you have time to move your mouth if you don't want to swallow. You can tap each other on the belly or back gently or more energetically as a signal to go slower or faster. Point your right forefinger to the right when you want your lover to move slightly to the right and move your left forefinger to the left when you want your lover to move slightly to the left.

Stick your thumb up in the "OK" sign to communicate "don't move," and clap your hands in a gentle applause to signify, "that it feels great."

Where to Come

Statistics show that 35 percent of men prefer to climax through oral sex rather than intercourse, but the question is, where do they like to climax? The number-one answer certainly is inside a woman's mouth. If you don't want to swallow, don't enjoy the taste of semen, but don't want to disappoint your man, here's a little trick that could save the moment. As soon as you get the sign that he's about to climax, whether he's tapping you on the shoulder or you feel his testicles rising, flip your tongue on top of his penis as opposed to keeping it under his penis. This will prevent his semen from spurting on to the side of your tongue where the majority of your taste buds are located. Keep your lips tightly wrapped around the head of his penis as you change the position of your tongue, and he'll never notice the difference.

Oral Info

Taste buds can be seen on the tongue as little red dots or raised bumps, particularly at the front of the tongue. Taste is also mainly a smell. If you hold your nose, close your eyes, and try to tell the difference between grated apple and grated onion, you can't. Try it.

An alternative is to let him come in your mouth and then discreetly spit his semen into a towel close by.

Some men like to watch their semen squirt, so they prefer to climax on a woman's face, breasts, tummy, or pubic mound.

If you don't want to experience his ejaculation on you, then move your mouth to his frenulum as he is climaxing so his semen will shoot toward his own stomach.

Lots of women are grateful for condoms because men ejaculate inside the condom, not inside or on top of them.

How to Get Him to Go Down

It's up to you to encourage the guy to go down south. Most guys don't have a clue, and many have to be hit over the head (figuratively speaking) to know that's what the girl wants. Here are some things to try.

A gentle "nudge." When the guy is kissing your breasts or stomach, you should do the same thing that that he often does: gently guide his head toward the land down under by pushing him there. He'll get the point.

Give feedback by making some noise. Moan like crazy! Scream. If you're afraid to scream because of the neighbors, then hold your hand over your mouth and try to scream. You'll still be releasing sexual and vocal energy, but you won't make as much noise. Let him know it's pleasurable as he gets closer, from breasts, to stomach, and so on … No guy will stop if he hears his efforts recognized. They all want to feel like studs. So humor them!

Talk dirty to him. "Eat me," "Lick me harder," "Flick your tongue softly on my clit," "Suck my lips as hard as you can and tickle my clit," "Finger my G-spot and suck my clit softly." Tell the guy what you want! Every girl is different. Don't make the guy guess!

If you like it hard with consistent rhythm, tell him. If you like it soft and sucked like a peach, tell him! No guy is a mind reader, and even if he's experienced, no two girls are alike.

Suggest a 69. Better still, just get on top of him in the 69 position and start giving him a blow job while you sit on his face. He's not going to have much choice, is he?

Watch porn. Show the guy how much you get off when a girl is being eaten properly.

Some guys simply aren't into it. For guys who don't like it, tease him with kisses and tastes of a flavored lubricant or gel and then put it on your clit and direct him to the strawberry or cherry flavor that you just exchanged with kisses. It's the idea of objectionable taste that freaks some guys out. Like sushi, it's an acquired taste for some ... and a matter of social upbringing and confidence for others. So for those who are pussies about eating pussy ... rope them in slowly, one lick at a time.

The Least You Need to Know

- Wetter is better because it's slippery, sexy, and succulent; use plenty of saliva when going down.

- To impress him, move your mouth as far down over his penis shaft as you can and suck slowly and deeply.

- Unless asked not to, handle his testicles lightly and lick them, then take each one into your mouth and suck gently making them all wet.

- To blow his mind, give him oral sex and hand combinations simultaneously.

Chapter 6

Basic Techniques for Him

In This Chapter

- Oral sex foreplay
- Techniques for stimulating her
- What to do with your hands during oral sex
- Basic positions for partaking in oral sex
- Get her to go down on you

In this chapter, you'll learn all the basics of oral sex foreplay as well as the essential moves for actually performing oral sex. You will also be introduced to different ways to stimulate her with your tongue. Then we move on to an explanation of some introductory positions for oral sex. Wondering about what to do with your hands? We'll go over what to do and where to put them as well. Then we'll end it all with a brief discussions on how to get your turn on the oral sex playground.

A Beginner's Guide to Worshipping the Vagina

Whether it's your favorite place, or you've never been quite face-to-face, the sooner you learn to worship her vagina, the better off you'll be. But don't go right for the end zone. You're going to need to create a game plan first.

Let the Games Begin

It may have been your idea, or it may have been hers. Either way, you're in the game now and it's time to perform. So where to begin? Unlike a lot of men, a lot of women want foreplay before oral sex. That isn't to say that some women don't want you to go right for the gold every time. However, to enhance your chances of success, it's best to start at the top. Kiss her lips, her neck, her breasts—get her really hot and bothered before heading south. As a matter of fact, it's best to make a road map of kisses as you work your way down. Don't forget her belly button! In a good game, tension mounts as you watch the play-by-play. The anticipation you create as you work your way down her body is sure to tease and arouse her even more.

The Long Way Around

All right, so you're heading toward the end goal, but something isn't quite right. It's that ugly four-letter word—*odor*. First of all, let me say this: The myth of the smelly vagina is just that—a myth. Perhaps, some fearful, lazy, selfish man who had no desire to please his partner concocted it and men who don't know any better continue to add fuel to the fire. But to say a vagina smells fishy is simply an exaggeration. All our body parts have the potential to be clean or dirty, malodorous or odor-free. The vagina is no exception. On the other hand, if you do go down on a woman who is emitting a strong scent, keep in mind this may be a sign that she has an STD or an infection. If that's the case, take this as a warning sign—Do Not Enter. Instead of using your mouth, consider using your hands to stimulate her vagina.

Assuming all things are healthy, if you run into the problem of odor, you may want to suggest to your lover that she take a shower. That doesn't mean you should give her a stinky complex while you're down in the trenches. Invite her to shower or take a bubble bath with you. Tell her you want to feel intimate with her before being sexual. Make it into a rewarding experience, not a punishment.

 Sexploration

The longest recorded orgasm was 43 seconds with 25 consecutive contractions. The record for the most orgasms by a woman in a single hour is 134.

Prefer a quick fix? All the major lubricant companies now manufacture flavored lubes in a variety of flavors. You're sure to find one you like. Apply a small amount to her clitoris, and you're in business.

Some people prefer the odor and taste of flavored lubes to the natural smell and flavor of their partner. Flavored lube may also decrease your partner's inhibitions about oral sex because she won't be worried about odors.

Getting There

Hopefully, you enjoyed going the long way around on your way down. You've completed your road map and arrived at your destination. Feeling nervous? So is she! So why not break the ice with something we all can feel good about—a compliment! Here's one that always goes over well: "You have the prettiest vagina." (Remember to read Chapter 1 for a discussion on what she wants you to call her vagina.) We all like to hear how attractive someone finds us, and that's not just from the waist up! Also, when you compliment her, you're helping her relax, which not only makes her feel better, it makes your job easier! A woman who feels confident and trusting is much easier to arouse than one who is feeling uptight and insecure.

A Man with a Slow Hand

Whoever said, "Patience is a virtue," was probably talking about her man in bed. True, desire comes in all shapes and paces, but it's safe to say a slow seductive hand can rarely go wrong. Besides, she'll tell you to speed it up when the time is right. Massage her labia (vaginal lips), gently running your finger along the seam where her lips come together. It may take a few minutes for you to get her really turned on and get her wet, so don't get discouraged. If you do this right, you'll probably inspire her to press herself into your hand, your wrist, your arm. This is a good thing! Once she's this turned on, you know she's ready for you to go all the way down.

Lick, Suck, Nibble, Caress

Now you're going to do with your mouth what you've been doing with your hand. Remember that road map of kisses? You're going to make a shorter one here, this time making lots of use of your tongue.

The Vulva

Kiss her mons (the soft area above her vagina that is covered with pubic hair or shaved of hair), working your way down from the top. The goal is not to miss a single place. If it helps, imagine you're kissing her face. Place delicate kisses where each cheek would be, where her eyelids would be, her forehead, her temples, her nose, her jaw, and her mouth. Continue until you've kissed the equivalent of her entire face. You may even want to give her a nibble here and there. Be sure not to bite too hard at first. If she asks for more pressure, don't be shy. Your job is to abide by her wishes. Now it's time to put that tongue to use. Run the flat of your tongue across her mons from bottom to top. Be sure you address both sides. You want to be sure she feels stimulated all over. After a couple minutes of kissing and licking, you can feel confident in moving on to the next step.

Outer Vaginal Lips

Trace the point of your tongue along the crease where her labia come together. Take one of her lips in your mouth and gently tug on it with your lips. Begin sucking, softly at first, building with her degree of excitement. You may even want to gently nibble on her labia. Alternately drag your teeth across her labia then suck. Nibble (gently) then lick. The variation in pressure and sensation will serve as a pleasant tease.

It's important to note here that some women absolutely lose their minds when you suck on their labia and some wonder why you're even wasting your time. So don't be put off if she doesn't respond. However, if she's one of those women who can't get enough, hop to it! She'd be more than happy for you to lick, nibble, and suck for a few minutes. Don't forget to repeat all that attention on the opposite side as well.

Inner Vaginal Lips

Working your way from outside in, you now find yourself at her inner vaginal lips. Hold her outer lips open with each hand as you press your mouth into her inner lips. Trace each side with the tip of your tongue, stimulating her with circular movements. Lick her from bottom to top with the flat of your tongue. Make your tongue dance around. Let your excitement add to and inspire her excitement.

Sexploration

The inner vaginal lips are more sensitive than the mons or the outer vaginal lips. Although everyone has her own preferences, biting here may prove rather painful for most. So you may not want to experiment with nibbling and love bites in this sensitive area unless she specifically asks you.

One Part Tease, One Part Follow-Through

Kiss her mons. Suck her labia. Run your tongue along the crease where her labia come together. Are you starting to feel like a tease? That's because you are one! But it's all right for you to tease if you can provide the follow-through. As she presses herself against you, slip your tongue inside her vagina, working your way up toward her clitoris.

The Final Touch

There are countless ways to stimulate a woman's clitoris. The important thing to remember is that she's in charge. Let her tell you whether she'd like it fast or slow, harder or softer, to the right or the left, up or down—you get my point! And if she's a little hesitant to instruct, ask. It makes no sense for you to work hard at something that isn't her thing.

Asking, "Baby, tell me what turns you on," is a turn-on in itself. It will cut down on her frustration and your own.

Now, having said all that, there are a few techniques you can keep in mind for stimulating her clitoris.

Simple Simon

The most basic cunnilingus technique is licking. A lot of people tend to use repetitive, quick, short strokes to the clitoris. There is nothing wrong with this technique, but there are other options as well. Use your entire tongue, dragging it across her clitoris from the base all the way to the point. Move your tongue from side to side like windshield wipers. Try circular motions as well, both around her clitoris and on it. Turn your head to the side, alternating again between licking in quick, short strokes and slowly dragging your tongue across her clit from base to point. Don't be afraid to come at her from a different angle!

You Suck!

A client of mine once told me a story about going down on a woman and having the feeling that he was doing nothing for her. Exasperated, he finally sat up and declared, "I suck!" "No, you don't," the woman replied. And that was a bad thing! She, as many women do, liked the feeling of having her clitoris sucked. Seem odd? Just think of it like a nipple. Wrap your lips around it and start sucking. The results are nearly immediate. She'll either swoon with delight or possibly flinch in pain. Don't let a flinch throw you completely off. She may just prefer you to suck more lightly as opposed to throwing in the towel altogether.

Mmmm, Mmmm, Mmmm

Mmmmmm—it's not just a sound, it's a sensation. That's right. What does a woman want to hear when you're between her thighs? That you're enjoying it! Sure, there are a variety of ways you can let her knows this, but here's why mmmm, mmmm is at the top of my list: Not only does it let her know you're enjoying the way she tastes, smells, and feels, but she will also be able to feel the vibration of the mmmm, mmmm, which is certain to arouse. And with two sources of pleasure, that's twice as much fun.

Tongue for the Masses

I had a friend who once told me he would sit in Mass as a child and, to kill time, he would flip his tongue over, rotating from left to right. This tongue flipping proved useful in his adult years. Now, don't fret if you've never been to Mass. This is a non-denominational technique everyone can master.

Start by practicing your tongue rolling by yourself in your down time. Practice in front of a mirror if you need to. When you're ready for the real deal, start by lining up the point of your tongue with her clitoris. As you spin your tongue, you will be essentially tracing the outside of her clitoris in alternating directions. This little maneuver is sure to win points. Once you have your sea legs, throw in a lick or a suck between rotations. Master this, and she'll be pulling out her hair—or yours!

Sexploration

If flipping your tongue over is something you can't even visualize, let alone master, don't lose hope! There are alternatives. Circle her clit with the tip of your tongue. Then change directions, and circle the other way.

Handy Work

All right, this may seem obvious, but it's worth saying. Don't forget you have hands—especially fingers! Whether you're kissing her vulva or licking her clitoris, your hands should never be at rest. Here are a few suggestions for how to keep them busy.

Massage

Begin by massaging her lower back while licking her vulva, inner labia, and clitoris. Work your way down, massaging, rubbing, and holding her behind. It's amazing how much more aroused a woman can get from being rubbed, held, or caressed in just the right place. It's your job to find out which of those places work best for the woman you're with. Then, be sure to massage and caress those places with your hands while you're licking, sucking, and nibbling with your mouth.

Take a Twist

Oral sex means using your mouth, but as we've already ascertained, that doesn't necessarily mean on her clitoris. Try licking her perineum (the area of skin between her anus and her vagina) while rubbing her clitoris with your thumb. Slip between your lover's legs. It may be easiest for her to bend one leg and for you to approach her from behind. Rest your head on her thigh as you run your tongue along her perineum, licking in long broad strokes. With the flat part of your tongue, lick her from the anus to the vaginal opening. Then, with the point of your tongue, trace zigzags across her perineum, like a skier doing the slalom. At the same time, rub her clitoris with your thumb. The combination of these two stimuli will send her through the roof. For an added twist, try the reverse. Lick and suck her clitoris while rubbing her perineum. This, too, is truly a winning combination.

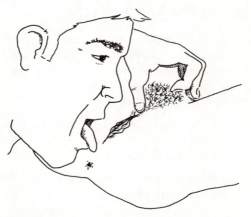

Thumb on clitoris, tongue on perineum.

The Finish Line

You've been massaging and licking for a while now.
By this point, she'll probably be begging you to
insert one or two fingers into her vagina. Be sure
your hands and fingers are clean first, then, go for
it. Again, she may prefer that you lick her clitoris
or her perineum. Either combination is a winner.
Insert your middle finger in slow motion first, and
then if she's very wet, insert your forefinger, too.

Sexploration

When a woman is close to reaching her
orgasm, you need to keep your tongue
and rhythm at the same pace and in the
same place. Don't change a thing until she
stops you.

Variety Is the Spice of Life

Who could ever count the wide variety of positions
in which we have sex? We all have our personal
favorites—along with our very own favorite varia-
tions. Oral sex should be no different. Here are a
few positions for you to brush up on:

Lazy Susan. She wants to lie on her back, and who
can blame her? Lie on your stomach between her
legs and set motion to her ocean.

Hanging Hannah. This position is similar to Lazy
Susan except she hangs her legs over the side of the
bed, and you kneel between them. At this angle,
you have greater access to more of her vagina.

Shoulder stance. This is Lazy Susan with a twist. She lies on her back. You kneel between her legs, and she raises her hips to you. You should help her hold herself up. If you're feeling strong, she may even throw her legs over your shoulders while you support her lower back. This isn't the easiest position to achieve, but it's fun for a little variety. And again, the change in the angle of your approach may stimulate her in unique ways.

Standing. This one's exactly as it sounds. She stands, you kneel. Be kind and give her something to lean on—a wall or a piece of furniture should do. Now, get to it. If you're any good at what you do, she'll need it!

Know When to Say When

You've touched. You've blown. You've coddled. You've grown old! Okay, not quite. But your neck hurts. Your face hurts. She's frustrated, and your tongue is about to go into spasms. In other words, you've been down there a while, and bursting volcanoes don't seem to be just over the horizon. That's okay. It's important to remember you can't hit it out of the park every time you step up to the plate. Ask her if there's another way you can please her. Or better yet, ask her if she'd like to please herself! Remember, it's not your fault. It's not her fault. There's no fault involved. Oral sex can be great even if it doesn't end with an orgasm. Enjoy the time you've shared together. And remember, there's always next time!

Watching Her

Most men love to look at women's bodies and that includes their genitals. Why do you think so many *Playboy*, *Penthouse*, and *Hustler* magazines sell each month? It's not for the articles. If you want her to pleasure herself in front of you, you have to help make her secure about the way she looks. Start by complimenting her face and body, then let her know how much she turns you on. Ask her to tease you by rubbing herself over her underwear first. If she's too uncomfortable to do that, she's not going to masturbate for you, so drop it.

If she agrees, reward her with more compliments as she caresses herself, then ask her to slide her panties to one side so you can see more. It's a good idea for you to pleasure yourself at the same time so she can watch your erection grow. Mutual masturbation is highly erotic and educational because you can watch each other stroke yourselves, and then learn how and where your lover wants to be touched.

Kissing Afterward

Some women love kissing after you've gone down on them, while others think it's gross. Start by kissing her breasts and work your way up to her neck, ears, and then around to her mouth. If she turns her head away or has a negative reaction, you'll sense it. Who knows? Maybe she'll pull your head up and give you a big smack on the lips herself. But don't forget, what's good for the goose is good for the gander.

How to Get Her to Go Down

Negotiate, barter, trade! It may sound silly, but it's the truth. In an ideal world, she'd want to go down on you just as much as you want to go down on her. (You do want to go down on her, right?) However, that's not always the case. For a wide variety of reasons she may not want to go down on you. The reasons can range anywhere from religion to hygiene to a bad experience—and everything in between. Getting to the bottom of the issue with your specific partner is at the heart of solving that problem, and I strongly encourage you to try. In the meantime, here is a list of some things to try to entice her to go down:

Look your best. If you want her to go down, keep your body clean and well groomed. Trim your pubic hair; better yet, shave your testicles. You know you like it when she is coiffed and sweet-smelling for you. Give her the same courtesy.

Show me the way. Go down on her first! This is an excellent way to break the ice. You may even be able to slip into 69 in the process. Or you may make her feel so fantastic she'll be begging to return the favor.

The devil's in the details. Okay, this is sad but true. Some women just aren't into sex, especially oral sex, as much as you. So offering to go down on her to inspire her to go down on you just isn't going to cut it. That doesn't mean you can't still negotiate, barter, and trade. You're just going to have to use a different currency. Figure out what she likes. It may be massages, going for picnics, dancing—you name it! It's your job to find out what pleases her so she'll want to please you.

Here are some hints for better communication around negotiating oral sex. Never say, "If you love me, you'll … (fill in the blank.)" Her reluctance to do something sexual is not a reflection on whether or not she loves you. Also, do not expect her to give you oral sex just because you gave it to her. It would be nice, but it isn't always the case. Be sure to express yourself clearly, honestly, and politely. You deserve to have your needs met, too!

The Least You Need to Know

- Taking your time to arouse her through some foreplay like kissing and caressing will make her more receptive to oral sex.

- Be sure your oral techniques include sucking the clitoris and licking the labia one after the other.

- Use your hands as an extension of your mouth on her breasts, stomach, inside of her thighs, buttocks, or vulva.

- Don't expect her to go down on you if you are not prepared to go down on her. You have to give to receive.

Chapter 7

Orgasms

In This Chapter

- Potential obstacles to reaching orgasm
- Your own pleasure scale
- The ultimate TriGasm
- Getting familiar fluids
- Female ejaculation

In this chapter, you'll learn how to create your orgasm pleasure scale. You'll discover the benefits of orgasms and understand what can prevent you from reaching an orgasm. There are lots of orgasms to choose from, and I'm going to share five of my favorite. Then it's onto the juicy subject of sex fluids like semen, saliva, vaginal fluids, and female ejaculation. In this chapter, there's even a recipe for a sex shake to make semen taste better.

What Is an Orgasm?

Orgasm is wired to our brain before it travels between our legs. It's a combination of emotional and most often, physical events that signal the brain to activate the body to experience involuntary physical responses, including:

- Increased breathing, additional blood flow to the genitals, and rapid heart rate
- Muscular contraction around the vagina, prostate, and anus
- The penis becoming erect and the vagina moist
- Men usually ejaculating as well as some women

Oral Info

Refer to the section on the male and female sexual cycles in Chapters 2 and 3 for more details on how an orgasm affects the male and female body.

So why are we seeking that euphoric, mind-blowing, earth-shattering, energy-melting orgasm? It is our second basic instinct after self-preservation (survival).

We also seek to lose that part of ourselves that connects us to the everyday and mundane. For a brief moment, we can lose the pain and hassle of being human and become one with the universe while we float on air like gods.

Orgasm Obstacles

If you have never experienced an orgasm you may be suffering from gynecological, urological, hormonal, or neurological disorders, so check with your medical practitioner first. If everything is in good working condition, then it's possible you have a psychological block such as one of the following:

- A traumatic past sexual experience
- Fear of losing control of yourself
- Resentment toward your partner
- Guilt about sex
- Fear of pregnancy
- Fear of intimacy
- Fear of failure or rejection
- Ignorance about your body's responses
- Lack of stimulation
- Low self-esteem and self-worth
- Inhibition

The good news is that you can get help to overcome these orgasm barriers from a professional sexologist, sex counselor, or therapist. Don't deprive yourself of orgasmic pleasure.

Your Orgasm Pleasure Scale

Imagine you have a personal pleasure scale ranging from number 1 to 10, with 1 being the minimum amount of arousal you can feel and 10 being the point of no return—orgasm! Now let's compare your pleasure scale to the Empire State Building, which has 102 floors. Picture the tenth floor as your number 1 on your pleasure scale and the 102nd floor as your number 10. There's a long way to go before you get to the reward of standing on the balcony and looking out at the beautiful view. Of course, some people will take the elevator and miss out on the experience of climbing 102 floors, while others will enjoy the journey and create anticipation of their arrival.

It's a good idea for everyone to recognize each level of arousal so they become familiar with how their body functions, discovering what turns them on the most. For example, getting a massage may only take you to a level 2 on your pleasure scale, whereas being kissed may take you to a level 4. Then masturbating may take you to a level 5, but mutual masturbation takes you to a level 6. Giving oral sex could take you to a level 7, and receiving oral sex may take you all the way to level 10. You are in control of your own pleasure scale, and you can learn a lot by watching your lover go up and down on his or her pleasure scale, too.

Take the time to create your personal pleasure scale and help your partner do the same. This is a wonderful exercise that will enhance your relationship in the communication, intimacy, and sexual department. Sexual knowledge results in sexual satisfaction!

Select Your Orgasm

There are many different kinds of orgasm you can experience from stimulation of different parts of your body. Each one will create different kinds of feelings, ranging from quick, short, localized, deep, concentrated, to full-body orgasms. This is your opportunity to experiment with as many different kinds of orgasm as you can. Remember, orgasm is good for your health, so it's doctors' orders!

A UniGasm

This is an orgasm resulting from stimulation directed to one primary erogenous zone such as the penis, prostate, testicles, clitoris, G-spot, anus, or nipples. In this example, I am going to focus on how nipple stimulation (for men and women) can produce an orgasm, though it's not as common as some of the other erogenous zones.

Oral Info

Did you know that for women, having their breasts caressed and nipples sucked releases oxytocin, the chemical that makes them feel like they are in love?

This is an area that many men enjoy stimulating during foreplay but rarely think of as having orgasmic potential. To give memorable oral sex on her breasts and nipples, you need to understand that the size of her breasts have nothing to do with the sensitivity. Ask her if she gets turned on by having her breasts played with. If so, then follow these directions.

Sexploration

To enhance oral nipple sensation, try putting an ice cube in your mouth while lavishing her orally.

Sexploration

As a woman, if you are not turned on by having your breasts or nipples played with, ask yourself why? If it's because you had an unpleasant experience with another lover, then put yourself in a new mind-set that that was then and this is now. If the idea is still unappealing, then guide your partner to another erogenous zone that does turn you on.

Begin by caressing and licking both of her breasts, not just her nipples. Alternate each one as you use the flat of your tongue in lapping motions all around her breasts, covering every centimeter. Follow your tongue with light fingertip caresses, saving her nipples until last. When both breasts are suitably wet from your tongue, cup your hand over one breast at a time so the tip of her nipple rests in between your thumb and your index finger. Squeeze your fingers together so you raise her nipple slightly and then begin licking it with the tip of your tongue in circular motions. After about a dozen or so lick, pucker your lips around the nipple and suck gently, but firmly, letting your head bob up and down simultaneously. Don't forget to give equal attention to both breasts and nipples. When she is climaxing, do not stop or change what you are doing. Let her push you away when she is ready.

For male nipple stimulation, the directions are pretty much the same, except men are more interested in having immediate nipple contact with deeper vacuum-sucking motions from the woman, not so much teasing around the nipple area. Some men even enjoy having their nipples nibbled on. So ladies, it's up to you to find out how much pain or pleasure your man wants on his nipples. Some men have one nipple that is more sensitive than the other. While you suck on one, you can pinch the other one and then ask him which one feels most erotic. You could be the first one to introduce him to a Uni-Gasm through his nipples. Now that's what I call creating a lasting mammary—I mean memory!

A BiGasm

Many people are experienced with various forms of dual stimulation—a penis and a tongue, a tongue and a finger, and the various other combinations. This will be more intense than a UniGasm, so it's worth exploring. Here are some ideal ways to create two points of stimulation.

It can be licking the testes while masturbating the penis, sucking on the clitoris while penetrating the anus with a finger (preferably covered with a finger cot), sucking the penis while massaging the testes, or licking the perineum while fingering the clitoris. Have fun experimenting with different combinations on your lover's body. Ask for feedback so you know which combinations are most exciting for him or her.

A TriGasm

So here's the revolution, the ultimate orgasm—a TriGasm. A female TriGasm is the result of arousing three points of pleasure—the clitoris, G-spot, and anus—simultaneously.

Here are some tips for you and your partner as you go off on your female TriGasm exploration:

Step 1: The woman should lie back while her partner lavishes her clitoris with oral pleasure until she has reached a level 8 on a pleasure scale of 1 to 10.

Step 2: Change course and stimulate her vulva (outside of the vagina) in small circles with your tongue for two minutes.

Step 3: Return to the clitoris and orally increase her level of pleasure to a 9, almost to the point of no return.

Step 4: At this peak, insert your forefinger palm up into her vagina and find her G-spot, then tap, tap, tap it gently toward her navel.

Step 5: Simultaneously with step 4, stimulate her anus gently with a feather, your pinky, or a vibrator to bring her to a momentous, energy-draining TriGasm!

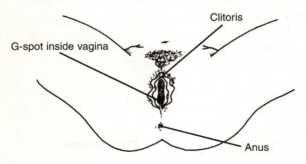

The female TriGasm.

The TriGasm for men is also the result of stimulating three points of pleasure—the penis, the testicles, and the anus—simultaneously:

Step 1: The man should lie back while his partner lavishes the head of his penis with some good oral suction until he reaches a level 8 on a pleasure scale of 1 to 10.

Step 2: Use your mouth and tongue to stimulate his testicles for two minutes while you masturbate his penis with your hand.

Step 3: Return to the penis orally and increase his level of pleasure to a 9, almost to the point of no return.

Step 4: For any kind of anal play, get plenty of lubricant ready. Saliva is not sufficient because it is too easily absorbed.

Step 5: At this peak, fondle his testicles as you continue to orally delight his penis and insert your forefinger palm up into his anus to find his prostate gland, then tap, tap, tap it gently. If all goes well, he'll have an unforgettable, enormous TriGasm!

Believe me when I say that you and your partner will not easily forget experiencing a TriGasm together.

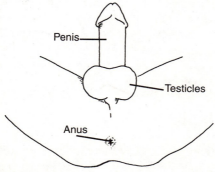

The male TriGasm.

A Blended Orgasm

A blended orgasm is exactly as it sounds, blending more than one orgasm. Start by choosing your favorite orgasm technique (such as oral stimulation on the clitoris for a woman and oral stimulation on the penis for a man). Get aroused to a level 6 on your pleasure scale and then switch to another orgasm technique you enjoy (such as G-spot for a woman and prostate for a guy) and get aroused to a level 7 this time. Switch back to the first technique, raise your arousal level to 8, then go back to the second technique at least three times before reaching a level 10 on your orgasm scale.

Multiple Orgasms

One definition of a multiple orgasm is when you reach one orgasm after another without any rest in between. Another definition is when you have an external orgasm and an internal orgasm simultaneously.

Do men have multiple orgasms? This is a controversial question, but I say, "Yes." When a man is able to separate ejaculation from his orgasm and he can remain sexually aroused at a very high peak, he can experience multiple orgasms much like a woman can. Multiple orgasms are a learned skill, and just about everyone can be taught to have them.

Sex Fluids

Sex is supposed to be wet and juicy; it can also sometimes be messy, as sex fluids like saliva, sweat, vaginal secretions, male ejaculate, and even female ejaculate all get mixed up together. Most people enjoy the wetness of sex because it implies that they are having a good time. When a woman's vagina becomes wet, it proves that she is sexually aroused; when a man has pre-ejaculate fluid oozing out of his penis, it means he's getting ready to ejaculate. It's important to enjoy your own body fluids and to accept your partner's wetness as part of the erotic sexual adventure that goes along with oral sex and lovemaking. The more you know about sex fluids, the more you can enjoy them, so I'm going to give you the basics on some of the natural fluids we produce when we're having sex.

Semen

Semen is created in the testes, where it takes about 10 weeks for a solitary sperm to reach maturity. The sperm can stay there for about two weeks before it's ready for ejaculation.

Semen contains more than 30 elements, including sperm, zinc, calcium, protein, enzymes, vitamin C, sodium, citric acid, fructose sugar, ascorbic acid, cholesterol, lactic acid, nitrogen, vitamin B_{12}, and various salts and enzymes.

The consistency of semen can vary depending on diet, medical problems, or even stress. When unhealthy, it can become thick or lumpy and the color can be greenish. The good news is that it has no impact on fertility, but don't delay a visit to your doctor for a check-up.

To maintain healthy semen, avoid smoking, alcohol in excess, coffee, and dairy products because these can make semen taste bitter. Drink plenty of water and eat fresh fruit.

Penis Talk

The approximate amount of semen per ejaculation is 1 to 2 teaspoons. With an average of 7 calories in a teaspoon of semen, it is not fattening. On the contrary, sperm is full of nutrition and protein; however, there's a chance you could catch an STD by swallowing.

To Swallow or Not To Swallow

Statistics show that 60.8 percent of men say that they want a woman to swallow their semen. These men admit this is a power play to prove that a woman will do anything for them. It's the ultimate display of trust. Other men don't care whether a woman spits out the semen or not after letting him climax in her mouth. However, my advice is that you should only swallow if you want to swallow. Don't ever let someone force or coerce you into doing something that goes against your personal values. There are always compromises like having the man ejaculate on a woman's face, over her breasts, or around her neck (known as a pearl necklace). It's still visually erotic for the man to watch and much less of a health risk for the woman.

Remember if you have oral sex without a condom, even if you don't swallow, it's possible to catch an STD, including HIV. Semen can contain all types of bacteria. The man you're having oral sex with could have an STD or HIV and not even know it.

Once the semen travels into the stomach, acids in the abdomen can kill the virus. But if there are any open cuts or wounds anywhere ahead of the stomach (including the mouth), there is a risk of infection.

Sexploration

If you want semen to taste its best, try this sex shake recipe formulated by Harley SwiftDeer: 2 teaspoon natural honey, 1 cup of milk, 1/4 teaspoon ground cinnamon, 1/4 teaspoon ground ginger, 1/4 teaspoon ground nutmeg, 1/4 teaspoon ground cloves, 1 raw egg. Put all the ingredients into a blender and drink one hour prior to oral sex.

Vaginal Fluids

Healthy vaginal secretion possesses high acidity as a natural resistance to bacteria and helps keep it clean. I've said it before, and I'll say it again: The vagina is the cleanest orifice in the body because it is self-cleaning and has a perfect pH balance. Vaginal fluids also keep the vagina moist and elastic.

In fact, throughout her monthly cycle, a woman's secretions can change in odor, texture, and color, especially during ovulation and her period. During ovulation, the secretions become much thicker and almost jellylike, and of course during her period her secretions are mixed with blood.

Vaginal secretions can potentially carry bacteria, fungus, and STDs. Unfortunately, antibiotics can cause a nasty discharge because they kill all bacteria, including good bacteria, which the vagina needs to function properly. It's important to learn the difference between healthy vaginal secretions and unhealthy ones. If there is a change in odor, the color turns yellow or green, or the texture is thick and crumbly, contact your gynecologist and get a check-up as soon as possible.

Saliva

Saliva comes from the salivary glands located inside of the cheeks and on the bottom of the mouth. These glands secrete slippery fluid every day of our lives.

Some of saliva's benefits include keeping our mouth relatively clean because it contains enzymes that help fight off infections (but brushing our teeth is still essential for oral hygiene). Saliva wets our food so it can push it toward the throat making it easier to swallow. Saliva also helps the tongue to taste and makes for a great natural lubricant when it comes to sex. Plenty of saliva on the head of a man's penis is an erotic way to begin oral sex.

However, as a sexual fluid, saliva can contain viral antibodies and STDs, so be careful not to kiss, lick, or suck someone if you or your partner have a cut or abrasion inside the mouth.

Can Women Ejaculate?

Some women are capable of ejaculating a fluid from their urethra during orgasm. This has been confirmed in several publications such as *The G-Spot and Other Recent Discoveries About Human Sexuality*, which offered the theory that a "uterine" orgasm (also known as a G-spot orgasm) can result in female ejaculation.

The fluid expelled looks like watered-down skim milk, and scientists describe it as having little or no color, taste, smell, or residue. The urethra is presumed to be the female prostate, so scientists have compared female ejaculation to male prostatic fluid, except without the sperm. The amount released varies from woman to woman from just a few drops to a gushing of liquid that can soak the sheets.

Any woman can learn to ejaculate, but not all want to. Some women associate it with loss of bladder control and are embarrassed that it might be urine. Although it is not urine, it's not as easy as men's ejaculation so not every woman has the desire to invest the time and effort into achieving it. Female ejaculation is associated with contractions of the pubococcygeus muscles during orgasm. These are also known as Kegels. Chapter 12 goes into step-by-step detail on how to do Kegel exercises. Also, Chapter 10 has instructions on how to stimulate the G-spot so a woman can learn to ejaculate if she wants to.

The most important thing to realize is that female ejaculation is a natural and healthy phenomena, so if you haven't tried it, what have you got to lose? Besides, 50 percent of men say they want a woman to ejaculate.

The Least You Need to Know

- Get to know your own arousal levels by imagining you have personal pleasure scale ranging from 1 to 10, with 10 being an orgasm.

- The ultimate orgasm is a TriGasm, stimulation of three points of pleasure simultaneously (the clitoris, G-spot, and anus or the penis, testicles, and anus).

- You can catch and spread STDs though sex fluids. This can happen when infected fluids are passed from one person to another.

- Women can ejaculate from their G-spot area when they are experiencing an orgasm; the amount of fluid varies from a few drops to more than a cup.

Chapter 8

Common Oral Sex Mistakes

In This Chapter

- Why you need to slow down
- Avoid some embarrassing and painful mishaps
- Find out what *not* to do with your mouth
- Don't underestimate the power of negative talk

From orally satisfying all your partner's erogenous zones to complimenting your lover's genitals, there are lots of oral rules you need to know before you can call yourself an oral master or mistress.

In this chapter, you will learn how to avoid some of the most common mistakes women make when handling the penis and men make when exploring the vagina. This chapter will explain why you shouldn't tackle the clitoris too soon and why you shouldn't neglect the testes when pleasuring the penis. You'll find out how to avoid oral pitfalls and make a good impression on your partner with some basic oral etiquette.

Don't Go South Too Quick

If you think there's only one way to give your lady the tongue down under, think again. But one of the first mistakes men make is going for the clitoris way too soon. Imagine if you're driving to the airport, you take the freeway to get there because it's quicker and more direct, right? But what if you're taking a drive for pleasure? Why wouldn't you take the scenic route and enjoy the drive? There's no hurry; you can take all the time in the world. Now doesn't that make you feel less pressured, more relaxed, and eager to drive?

Women really appreciate a slow driver when it comes to sex. They need time to get their juices flowing. Unlike most guys, who can get an erection at a moment's notice, women need to be prepared for sex, even oral sex.

If in Doubt, Leave It Out

The vagina is the cleanest orifice in the body because it's self-cleaning, unlike the mouth, which you have to keep clean by brushing your teeth, gargling with mouthwash, and even scraping and spraying your tongue free of bacteria. If you're good to the vagina, it will return the favor tenfold. So to keep you in its good graces, here are some things not to put inside a vagina:

Don't put small objects like marbles inside because they can get lost. The vagina is a large muscle designed to pull things in.

Don't rub or insert anything sugary like honey inside the vagina because it will upset the perfect pH balance that keeps it so clean and healthy. So no Popsicles, chocolate bars, or phallic fruit, either. If you must insert a banana, keep the peel on and put a condom on it first.

Don't insert anything oily because that will cause a nasty vaginal infection. So keep out Vaseline, baby oil, suntan oil, and all cooking oils. Lubricant is all right, as long as it's water soluble.

Don't blow smoke or even air inside the vagina because it can cause an embolism, which is an air bubble that can be fatal if the woman is pregnant.

Don't forget to remove tampons before intercourse because they can get lodged way up there and may have to be surgically removed.

Don't leave your fingernails jagged. Keep them neatly filed because they can cut the vagina.

Don't insert bottles or any other glass, which can shatter.

 Oral Info

Never put anything unsanitary inside the vagina, and that includes unclean fingers.

Don't put alcohol in the vagina. I know some people like to drink and then squirt a little booze into the vagina while giving oral sex. Alcohol will burn the delicate mucous membrane tissue of the vagina. This goes for all kinds of alcohol: wine, whiskey, brandies … everything.

If you don't put anything unsanitary inside her, she'll be happy, healthy, and horny. Always remember, if in doubt, leave it out!

No Bones About It

Regardless of what the penis is called when it's hard, the human penis does not have a bone in it. The penis is made up of spongy tissue surrounded by a fibrous cover that fills up with blood when aroused, creating an erection. Don't be afraid or intimidated by his erection, ladies; make him your user-friendly toy. Remember how excited you used to get when you were young and you received a new toy? I bet you looked at it, examined it, and played with it for hours. Make your man's penis your favorite toy, and turn sex into adult play!

Most men agree that they like more pressure on their penis than women like on their clitoris, but they'll wince if you squeeze too hard. So take his pride and joy in both hands, wet it with your saliva, and become familiar with it before you take it in your mouth. Don't ever masturbate your man's penis when it's dry; the friction could cause scratches and abrasions. Focus on moving his skin up and down— rather than moving your hand up and down.

Look at his penis admiringly, and feel free to compliment it out loud. Touch it, stroke it, tickle it, pump it between your palms, and rub it all over your body lovingly. A man likes to feel that his partner is enthusiastic about his penis before he surrenders it to her control.

Sexploration

If your man is circumcised, he probably enjoys extra stimulation around the visible scar tissue, located around the head of his penis. Go ahead and add some extra suction around that area as you give him oral sex.

Swallow This

Speaking of control, ladies, if you don't want to swallow, then tell your man before you start giving him oral sex, because he can't read your mind. Furthermore, he may not be able to control himself from climaxing when you're giving him oral sex. It's no fun when you're on the verge of an orgasm and your partner suddenly stops giving you oral sex!

Avoid being uncomfortable by talking to him about your sexual concerns before you become intimate. Voice any fears you may have about gagging or swallowing. Don't ever feel pressured into doing something you don't want to do. A good tip is to agree on a signal he can give you before he's going to climax—such as patting you on the shoulder twice.

Don't Forget the Testes

One of the biggest complaints I hear from men is that their lovers neglect their testicles. My advice to men is to remove the hair from their testicles so women will find them more palatable. The penis and testicles are connected, and the penis shaft extends down behind the testicles. Both the penis shaft and the testicles deserve equal attention. It's like putting lipstick on your upper lip and leaving the lower lip without any color.

The testicles are one of the most sensitive parts of the male sexual organ. Touch his testicles delicately, as if you were handling a light bulb. Go ahead and feel, caress, and fondle them, but don't squeeze them too hard. You can also handle the scrotum without touching the testicles; it's less sensitive, but equally erotic and satisfying for the man.

Most men enjoy a wet mouth and talented tongue around their balls, so get used to sucking on the scrotum first and gently tugging on them with your lips, not your teeth. Then take one testicle at a time into your mouth and suck ever so gently, as if you were sucking on a soft-boiled egg, carefully trying not to damage the yolk. After that, suck both testicles at the same time.

Getting Down

Now here's one for the guys: Please don't push her head down onto your penis while she's sucking it unless she tells you that she likes it. It turns off some women because it makes them feel like they are being forced to give you oral sex.

However, feel free to run your fingers through her hair and gently pull her hair off her face so you can watch her give you oral pleasure. Caress her face tenderly, and give her plenty of encouragement by letting her know how good she makes you feel. The more you tell her that she's skillful, the more she'll want to please you.

Ejaculating Too Quick

How does it make you feel when your sexy lover goes down on you? She begins to lick the head of your penis with her luscious tongue, parts her lips and takes your shaft deep into her mouth, and then suddenly it's all over—you couldn't hold back and you came much sooner than you wanted. Some men say it makes them feel inadequate as a lover; others just get mad at themselves. Premature ejaculation can happen to anyone, but if want to avoid the embarrassment, here are some precautions you can take:

- If you haven't had sex in a long time, masturbate about four hours before your planned encounter.

- If you are getting oral sex and you feel like you're going to climax, ask the woman to stop. Then give her oral sex for a while.

- You can squeeze the base of your penis when you feel like you're going to climax too early.

There are more detailed exercises in Chapter 12 that can help with premature ejaculation and maintaining an erection.

Common Turn-Offs

Here are some things to keep in mind before you get busy:

Don't attack your lover's sense of smell by pouring on too much perfume or cologne, especially around your genitals. There's nothing sexier than the aroma of a clean body. Even if it cost you a small fortune, go easy on the perfume—it tastes bad, it can linger on the sheets and furniture, and it can even cause allergies.

Don't put talcum powder on your genitals before oral sex because it clumps up when you sweat, looks yucky, and tastes horrible.

Don't use depilatory cream to remove pubic hair just before getting oral sex. The skin is very sensitive after using depilatory cream, and even a wet tongue can result in a burning sensation. The odor also lingers for several hours. It's best to use the cream the night before.

Don't, and I mean, *don't* leave a hickey as your calling card on your lover unless he or she asks you to.

Teeth Don't Cut It

Whether your teeth brush up against a penis or a clitoris, it will spoil the moment and possibly the rest of the night. Most of the time, if your teeth come in contact with your partner's skin, you probably won't realize it, but your partner will!

For her: The first step to keeping your teeth off his penis is to be *aware* that you have sharp weapons in your mouth. The next step is to be sure your jaw is open relatively wide when giving oral sex so your teeth won't come in contact with your partner's genitals. In the heat of passion, to avoid accidental scraping, wrap your lips around your teeth. Ladies, this is especially important when you are *deep-throating* your man. If you are still unable to control your teeth, another alternative is to cover them with plastic teeth guards that come in over-the-counter teeth-whitening kits.

Penis Talk

To **deep-throat** someone is a form of oral sex in which the penis is voluntarily taken deeply into the recipient's throat.

For him: The worse thing a guy can do is to chew on the clitoris. No wonder some women resort to faking their orgasms! Start licking the clitoris gently with the tip of your tongue. As you feel her thrusting forward, keep your upper lip over your teeth to protect her from getting bitten, and continue licking with rhythmic stokes. She will continue to push her lower body toward you in her desire for more pressure, and all you have to do is to continue licking until she pushes you away.

Dry Mouth

There's nothing worse than having a dry mouth when you are trying to satisfy your partner orally, so try to have a near by glass of water so you can take a discreet sip whenever you need it. If you're feeling adventurous, add some ice cubes to use on your lover for some sensual foreplay. The same goes for a towel or tissues to wipe away body fluids. Keep them close by so you don't have to jump up as soon as you and your partner have climaxed. Some people prefer the taste of flavored lubricants to the natural taste of their partner's genitals, so keep these handy if you're going to use them.

It's bad etiquette to get up in the middle of adult play to get a glass of water or even to go to the bathroom. It breaks the mood. Go to the bathroom before you make love. Open up your condom, get out your sex toys, and prepare everything you need before you get all worked up. Better still, go to the bathroom together and take a shower or bubble bath before oral sex so you both feel squeaky clean.

What Did You Say?

When you're giving or receiving oral sex, here are some things you definitely don't want to say:

Don't talk about problems. It's a sure way to kill the mood, and it lets your partner know you're not turned on.

Don't talk about your body negatively. Don't blurt out, "I wish my stomach was flatter." Worse still, don't insult your partner's body.

Don't compare your partner to anyone else you have slept with.

Don't call her a whore or anything else that is derogatory, unless you both discuss it beforehand. Some women enjoy hearing sexually graphic language while they are giving fellatio. So if your lover gives you permission to talk to her like a whore, then by all means, go for it—just don't assume its okay.

Don't ask a woman if she came. You should know whether she did or not by her body language. For more information on a woman's orgasm, review Chapters 3 and 7.

Don't ask your lover to answer an awkward question like, "Am I the best lover you've ever had?" especially if you can't handle the truth.

Don't say "Stop" when you mean "Go," and don't say "No" when you mean "Yes."

Don't negatively express directions to your lover on how you like to receive oral sex. It's okay to say, "I love it when you lick the head gently with your tongue," but it's not okay to say, "Why don't you lick the head more?"

Don't get carried away during oral sex and say something you'll regret later like, "I love you," if you don't mean it. Instead, you can say, "I love making love to you," or "I love being with you," but don't ever play with someone's emotions.

Sexploration

There are two very powerful words you can use in bed that will turn on your partner. The first one is "yes," and the second is his or her name. Use them often ... and be sure you say the right name.

The Least You Need to Know

- The vagina is the cleanest orifice in the body, so don't put any food or anything unsanitary inside it because it will upset its perfect pH balance.

- Ladies, play with and have the same enthusiasm for your lover's penis as if it was your favorite new toy.

- The penis and the testicles deserve equal attention by being caressed, licked, and sucked.

- Do not chew or bite on the clitoris unless she asks you to. It has 8,000 nerve fibers and its very sensitive, so start out gently.

Chapter **9**

Oral Sex Options

In This Chapter

- Improve technique through new positions
- Have fun with sex toys
- Find out if back door stimulus is for you

Now that you know some basic oral sex techniques, it's time to turn up the heat with various oral sex options. By the time you've finished this chapter, you will be well on your way to becoming an oral master or mistress.

In this chapter, you'll discover how to incorporate some common household items into foreplay and why sex toys have therapeutic value. You'll have the opportunity to expand your sexual horizon by sharing your sexual fantasies and role-playing with your lover. Enjoy legendary aphrodisiacs, and for the truly adventurous, embark on some back door fun.

Positions for His Pleasure

Receiving oral sex feels great in pretty much any position you choose, and there are lots to select from. Some positions make you feel more outgoing than others, and each position stimulates you differently. I encourage you to try new positions and locations if you want to maintain excitement in your sex life.

Contented Male Position #1

All guys love this position—all they have to do is lie on their back with a pillow under their head and another pillow under their buttocks. This position can be accomplished on a bed, a couch, or the floor. It offers easy access to his penis, testicles, and anus and allows him to lie back totally relaxed. Ladies, you can rest yourself in between his legs, on your stomach so you have a bird's-eye view of his entire genital area.

Begin by taking his penis in your hands and licking the head in circular motions as you maintain eye contact with him. Apply plenty of saliva to make his penis wet and slippery. Next, wrap your lips tightly around the head of his penis (glans), and use your mouth as a vacuum (not an industrial vacuum—more like a handheld vacuum), by lavishing him with ample suction.

Now you are well on your way to giving him a memorable blow job, so don't forget to incorporate all the lessons you learned in the basic oral sex techniques. Remember to make sounds of pleasure as you orally delight him, use your hands as an extension of your mouth, and don't forget to stimulate his testicles.

Contented Male Position #2

The lucky guy stays in the same position as in "Contented Male Position #1," but ladies, you get to sit on his chest, facing away from him. If you lift your buttocks up slightly, it will give him an erotic visual of you, while you have a new angle for orally pleasing him. If you suffer from the gag reflex, this angle will help lessen it. It's also a great position for you to stimulate his prostate area.

Contented Male Position #3

The guy remains on his back, lifts his knees to his chest, and places his feet on his lover's shoulders while she kneels between his legs. His penis, testicle, and anus are on complete display, giving her easy access to do what she does best.

Let's Face It

She is lying on her back. He puts his knees on either side of her face so his penis hovers over her mouth. He can do this facing her or facing away from her. Either way, she gets a good angle for some deep throating. Communicate in advance if you want him to remain still while you move your head and hands or if you want him to thrust his penis in and out of your mouth. This angle is also great for orally pleasuring the testicles and the anus. (We'll expand on analingus a little later in the, "Back Door Fun" section.)

Doggie Pose

It's nice to know that this position is conducive to more than just intercourse. It's actually a great angle for receiving oral sex, both for men and women. Let's focus on his pleasure first as he gets into doggie pose on his hands and knees with his legs spread apart. By drawing his penis back between his legs, he can now be lavishly licked and sucked by his partner.

Instead of getting on your hands and knees, try bending him over a bed, chair, or even a table and use the furniture as leverage instead of putting all the weight on his hands and knees. If you want to be even more comfortable, just lie down on your stomach with your legs spread wide apart. Your partner can still get a mouthful of your penis and testes. Remember, variety is the spice of life, and that includes oral sex positions.

Positions for Her Pleasure

Receiving oral sex for a woman is one of the great wonders of the world. Getting into various oral sex positions is an added enjoyment she will be only too happy to engage in, especially when she is the focus of attention.

Contented Female Position #1

Now it's the lady's turn to lie back comfortably with a soft pillow under her head and another under her buttocks. Raising her pelvis with a pillow will provide him with the best access to her clitoris, vagina, and anus. It will also help alleviate strain from his neck. In this classic position, keep your legs spread flat on the bed so he can lie between them. Use your hands to stroke his hair and gently guide his head in the right direction. Guys, feel free to put your arms under her legs so you can draw her buttocks even closer to you. Don't squeeze her cheeks too hard, but spread them apart gently. Now enjoy giving as much as you did getting.

Contented Female Position #2

Still lying on your back, raise both legs and rest them on your lover's shoulders. This position is one that gives your sexual organs full exposure and even better oral access. Some women like it when their lover lifts their buttocks up high, but be careful because it can put a strain on her back as it arches up. For others, the pleasure outweighs the discomfort.

Contented Female Position #3

Ladies, you are still the receiver of oral pleasure so remain on your back, and bend and raise your knees so you can rest them on his chest. Now surrender yourself to his mouth and tongue.

Let's Face It

Straddle his face by squatting or kneeling over him. Wear a G-string, and pull it to one side to tease him first.

You can face him or turn the other way. Either way, it's a great oral sex position for the woman because she can control the pressure and tempo of the pleasure she is getting. By lifting and lowering the vagina, grinding the hips, and tilting the pelvis, she's in control.

Doggie Pose

This position is particularly popular with women who are sexually uninhibited. Licking her from behind while she's in doggie pose gives the man great access to her vagina and anus. Men find this position one of the most erotic, and women love the stimulation they get from this angle.

Instead of getting on your hands and knees, try bending over a bed or some furniture you can use as leverage instead of putting all the weight on your hands and knees. If you want to be even more comfortable, just lie down on your stomach with your legs spread wide apart. This position is great because you can stimulate your clitoris while your lover lavishes oral sex on and in your vagina. Be prepared to reach your climax sooner than you think.

Sit On It

Sit upon your throne and prepare to be orally pampered. Actually, you can sit anywhere—on the edge of the bed, on the kitchen counter, or even on the tumble dryer—which is best when it's on spin cycle. Your lover will kneel or crouch in front of you, and he'll either hold your legs up over his head or let them rest on his shoulders. Either way, you'll be the receiver of oral delights.

Stand for It

This is a hot fantasy for both sexes. Ladies, this is your opportunity to dominate your man. Stand up against a wall or counter and ask your lover to kneel down before you. Lift one leg and put your foot on his shoulder. Watch out for the high heels. Now hold on to his head and guide it toward your vagina while you give him plenty of encouragement.

The Versatile Sixty-Niner

A sixty-niner is a great position for mutual oral sex. First you have to decide who is going to be on top—my suggestion is the lighter one of the two of you should be on his or her hands and knees over the other. Admittedly, it can be distracting when you're trying to give oral sex and you're receiving it at the same time. Be careful not to get too aggressive with your lover's genitals in this position. If you have trouble keeping rhythm or concentrating on giving while you're receiving, you can stay in the sixty-niner position and masturbate your partner while she or he is giving you oral sex. Here are a couple more options:

Sixty-Niner Sideways: This position is most comfortable for people who are of ample weight, which includes pregnant women. Lie down on your side, your mouth facing your partner's genitals. Because your head is in between your partner's legs, you can use each other's thighs as a pillow.

Sixty-Niner Standing: This is only for the truly athletic, not for the weak at heart. Lift up your lover and spin her around so her vagina is in your face and her head is down between your legs so she can put her mouth around your penis. Now hold on to her nice and tight because you don't want to drop her on her head. This position is as advanced as you can get, and it's also very playful. Just give each other a few good licks and then put her back down the right way up. Though it's not a great position to reach orgasm, I guarantee it will be memorable.

Talk to each other about which positions you enjoy the most and why you find them more exciting than others. By changing positions during oral sex, the receiver experiences a variety of feelings according to the angle.

Lick Around the House

Now that you've learned some new oral sex positions, it's time to change locations. Whether you live in a house or an apartment, there are several options to choose from. Christen every room in your home by having an orgasm in each one.

You don't want to always make love in the same old place, in the same old position at the same old time—boring, boring, boring! There's no better way to keep your love life fresh than to keep your lover guessing, "I wonder where we'll make love next."

Toys Are for Adults, Too

A sex toy is anything you use to enhance foreplay or sex. Now that you've made love in every room, it's time to find as many common household items as you can to enhance sensual pleasure. Here are some clues: a feather duster, rolling pin, ruler, spatula, hair brush, telephone, flashlight, pillows, toothbrush—need I go on?

The most commonly used sex toy is the vibrator. Many people think of vibrators as a woman's tool to be used for solo pleasure during masturbation. However, many men enjoy the stimulation of a vibrator on their genitals, testicles, and anus. And of course couples can incorporate vibrators and other sex toys into their lovemaking.

Oral Info

Don't forget to clean your sex toys with soap and water as you would anything else you use regularly. You can also practice putting condoms on the vibrators and dildos for fun.

I believe sex toys have therapeutic value because they can help people overcome inhibitions, add a wonderful source of variety, and can spice up a predictable lovemaking session. They can also take performance pressure of the man and help both sexes to reach orgasms more readily. And of course the sex toy can keep on going and going as long as it has working batteries. Today there are hundreds of vibrators and dildos in all shapes and sizes. I recommend couples go sex toy shopping together so they can each pick out one sex toy they want to take home with them. Whether you visit a sex toy shop or purchase your adult toys on the Internet, you'll have something new and exciting to add to your sexual repertoire. A word of caution: Never use a sex toy for the vagina, that has been inserted into the anus and never share your sex toys with anyone else.

By combining vibrators and dildos with oral sex, you can fantasize that you're having sex with more than one person and add extra stimulation at the same time.

For her: Imagine you are lying back, enjoying the way your lover is licking your clitoris and he's slowly penetrating your vagina with a realistic dildo at the same time. You can fantasize that you have two lovers; you can experience a clitoral orgasm and a G-spot orgasm simultaneously and enjoy the uninhibited pleasure of surrendering yourself to your partner.

For him: Visualize your lover is straddled above you in the sixty-niner position as she is giving you a phenomenal blow job. Your erect penis is filling her mouth—then she takes a vibrator and places it in the middle of your testicles. You are experiencing suction around your penis, vibration in the center of your testicles, then ... she adds a vibrating butt plug to the opening of your anus. The feeling is unbearably good, and you can't hold back anymore. You're in sex toy heaven.

Back Door Fun

Many people wince at the thought of anal play because they consider the anus an exit, not an entrance, and certainly not a lickable source of power-packed pleasure. For others, though, rimming, or analingus (kissing, caressing, or penetrating the anal opening with a tongue) is an orgasmic experience. Because many consider the anus taboo, it can heighten the erotica both for the giver and receiver. The anus is surrounded by sensitive nerve endings, which is another reason why it can take you to the point of no return.

Great oral sex can include stimulating the anus with a feather, vibrator, pinky, or tongue. Here are some anal tips for the anal adventurer:

- The easiest position for rimming or analingus is doggie pose.

- Start by gently kissing your partner's butt cheeks.

- Using the flat of your tongue, lick your partner's perineum (located between the man's testicles and his anus or the woman's vaginal opening and her anus) all the way to your partner's anus.

- With the tip of your tongue, lightly lick around the anal button in circular motions.

- With a pointy tongue, give your partner's anus an in-and-out massage.

As a word of caution, you should know that the anus is not as clean as the vagina. In fact, it is filled with bacteria so oral-anal contact is not a safe one. Unprotected, it can transmit viruses that include HIV, hepatitis, herpes, and warts. Always use a barrier such as a dental dam or even transparent food wrap.

The Least You Need to Know

- Have oral sex in a variety of positions, and discuss which ones you enjoy the most.

- Don't always have oral sex in the same place. Add spice to your sex life by doing it in every room in your home.

- You don't always have to purchase sex toys. Any object you use for sexual enhancement (such as a common household item) automatically becomes a sex toy.

- Oral-anal contact is unsafe unless you use a barrier like plastic food wrap or a dental dam over the anus before putting your mouth and tongue on or in it.

Chapter 10

How to Rock Her World

In This Chapter

- Stimulate her senses
- Give her a tongue massage
- Put more bliss in a kiss
- Go on an expedition to find her goddess spot

In this chapter, you'll get the facts on what women need to be fully aroused. You'll learn how to stimulate all her senses, get the lowdown on how to identify your lover's erogenous zones with your tongue, learn tips on facial intercourse and shrimping, and understand why enthusiasm is so important. You will feel like a hero when you discover her goddess spot and help her achieve multiple orgasms. This chapter will help create the most memorable sex of her life.

Scentsational Sex

The number-one reason you choose a lover above anything else is because you love the way they smell. Our natural pheromones are how we attract our mates. These pheromones come from our sweat glands that are attached to our hair follicles. So wherever there is hair, there are pheromones: in our scalp, under our arms, and in our pubic hair.

Pheromones are released into the air from sweat that evaporates from our skin in the 40 million skin cells we shed each day.

Oral Info

If you don't use one of your five senses during lovemaking, you miss out on 20 percent of pleasure.

Smell This

Our most powerful sense is smell, because smell receptors in the nose are directly wired to the limbic center of the brain. It controls our sex drive, emotions, and sensual memories. So a smell can arouse us, trigger an emotion, or evoke a memory.

If you want to rock her world, you need to know how to heighten all her senses. I can tell you that women are attracted to the aroma of musk, orange-blossom, and sandalwood, many of which are ingredients found in men's cologne. So before buying any, ask her what kind of men's fragrance turns her on. Food aromas that turn women on include melon, chocolate, oranges, and fresh bread. You can also stimulate her sense of smell with scented candles, fresh flowers, or incense.

What a Sight

We all know how visual guys are, which is why they love to see their ladies wear sexy lingerie. But don't underestimate your woman's sense of sight. She wants to be stimulated visually just as much as you do. Women love to see their man perfectly groomed, so always try to look your best for your lover. Arouse her sense of sight by lowering the lights or candlelight and give her oral sex in front of a mirror. Some women love watching erotica, too—I have a feeling you won't object if she wants to watch an adult movie with you.

I Hear You

Nothing stimulates the sense of hearing better than some erotic talk. Whisper lots of compliments in her ear and tell her how you plan to seduce her orally. Don't forget to use her name. Other sensual sound stimulants are a crackling fireplace, music, nature sounds, and even the sounds of other people making love. You can always record yourselves having sex and then play it back the next time you make love.

Touch Down

Slowly, sensuously undress your lover and caress, kiss, and lick every part of her body as you peel off her clothes. Give her oral sex on satin sheets; caress her body with different fabrics like feathers, silk, velvet, or leather. Cover her body in massage oil, lotion, or powder. Just don't touch that TV remote, because she should be the one and only focus of your attention.

Taste Me

Prepare some erotic finger foods in advance of your sexual activity. Feed each other and lick each other's fingers before moving south of the border. Use edible lotions, potions, and lubricants, but remember to put these foods and products on your lover, not inside her vagina because it has a perfect pH balance that should not be upset.

Lick Her from Head to Toe

How many times have you heard that women want foreplay, and plenty of it? Well, I'm here to confirm that it's true. We need to be prepared for sex to get our natural juices flowing. One of the most effective ways to get us in the mood for love, especially oral love, is for you to stimulate, our erogenous zones. We are covered in erogenous zones (places on the body that, when stimulated give us, pleasure and lead to sexual arousal) from head to toe. It's your job to discover our primary erogenous zones and then work us up to a sexual frenzy.

The best way to discover your lover's erogenous zones is to kiss and lick her from her head to her toes in slow motion. Don't leave out any areas, especially if you see an imperfection like a mole or a scar. Go ahead kiss the flaw on her body. It will help her relax and give her more sexual confidence. Now ask your lover to rate her erogenous zones on a pleasure scale from 1 to 10 with 10, being orgasmic. You can use your tongue to help her discover new, exquisite zones of pleasure. Wet your tongue;

use it dry; try circular motions; sweeping motions, and spell your name on your lover's body. This will prepare you for more advanced oral sex techniques later on.

Facial Intercourse

Kissing is so intimate and erotic that I like to call it facial intercourse. The way you kiss also reveals a lot about the way you give oral sex. Most women love to be kissed for at least five minutes. Pay attention to her face before you go below the belt. Add some variety to your standard kissing technique. Start by brushing her hair back off her face and gently massage her scalp as you cover her face with baby kisses.

Then lick her upper and lower lips with the tip of your tongue. Now run your tongue over her teeth. Wrap your lips around her tongue and suck deeply and gently, then dart your tongue in and out of her mouth and let her tongue search the inside of your mouth. Your journey has only just begun.

Sexploration

There are lots of different kinds of kisses: slow, quick, wet, dry, long, etc. Don't take the art of kissing for granted. Add variety to your kissing technique and make it last for a minimum of 12 seconds.

Now that your tongue is all warmed up, it's time to explore all her erogenous zones. Remember to get feedback from her on which ones turn her on the most. You don't need to write them down, but you do need to remember the ones that are rated 8 and above.

- Kiss her ear lobes gently. If she rates it a high number, continue to kiss, lick, and suck on them. She'll start to turn to putty in your hands.

- Massage her neck and shoulders with your fingertips, and follow with quick flicks of your tongue.

- The fingers are especially sensitive. Spread two fingers apart at a time and lick in between them with a pointy tongue.

- Here's one I bet you didn't know. The armpits are an erogenous zone for many women—so give it a lick and find out if your lover is one of them.

- The breasts are an obvious hot spot, and they should be kissed and fondled gently. Avoid contact with the nipples until after you've kissed and licked the underside of her breasts. A common criticism I hear from women is that men are too rough with their nipples. If you start out by kissing, licking, then sucking the nipples softly, you can't go wrong.

- A woman's belly is all too often neglected by traditional massage therapists, so here's your chance to lightly tickle her belly, followed by light circular licks with your tongue.

- Inside the thighs are especially responsive to a nice wet tongue—tease her inner thighs without touching the genitals.

- Ask her to turn over and lick the back of her neck, then blow your warm breath on her nape and shoulders.

- Licking up and down the spine can create goose bumps, so wet your whistle and go for it.

- Her buttocks are just aching to be massaged, kissed, and licked.

- Slide your tongue up and down the back of her thighs—if your tongue gets tired, alternate kisses and licks.

You've invested some quality time exploring your lover's feminine curves. You're on your way to "rocking her world"—the more you tease her, the more excited she'll become and the quicker she'll climax.

Shrimping

Before you focus on her vagina, there's one more area that needs particular attention. Her toes! Having her toes licked is a major turn-on for some women. Be sure you give every toe equal attention by licking in between each one and then sucking them individually. This is a popular fetish known as shrimping. It's fittingly named because the toes on your feet resemble a row of shrimp.

Don't Curb Your Enthusiasm

I've said it before, and I'll say it again, "Enthusiasm is more important than technique." Fortunately for you, this book will help you with both. Women love a man who is enthusiastic, especially when it comes to giving her oral sex. The more you let her know how much you love going down on her, the better. Tell her that she tastes delicious, she smells great, and her vagina looks beautiful. Let her know that you could give her oral sex all night long, if that's what she wanted.

Do the Alphabetti

This technique will take your lover to the point of no return and back again. Just let her know that she is going to be the receiver of pleasure and you are going to be the giver. I hope you can remember the alphabet because you're going to spell it out on her vagina with your tongue. If all goes according to plan, she'll have the big "O" before you even get to O.

The best position for this is any of the contented female positions (from Chapter 6) where she is lying comfortably on her back with a pillow behind her head and another under her buttocks.

1. Start by covering her vagina with your entire mouth. This lets her know she's in for a treat. Incidentally, I recommend that you end each oral sex session with the same loving ritual by covering her entire vagina with your entire mouth for a few seconds.

2. Now begin tracing the capital letter A with the tip of your tongue from the top of her clitoris all the way down to the opening of her vagina. Make your tongue flat and wide when you cross the letter A.

3. The letter B has a few more curves in it, which will stimulate different parts of her vagina. Use a firm tongue stroke to circle the top of the B around her clitoris, inadvertently flicking it before you tongue the second circle.

4. Continue to slide and twist your tongue around her vulva as you spell the rest of the alphabet.

Use your tongue in different ways, alternating from up and down, side to side, small and big circles, soft and firm, quick and slow, pointed and flat. Have a good time exercising your tongue and pleasing your mate. I'm betting she won't let you finish the alphabet. Incidentally, you can also trace numbers on her vagina.

Where Is the Goddess Hiding?

The G-spot, which I like to refer to as the goddess spot because it makes us feel like a goddess when it's stimulated, is not a myth—every woman has one, though not every woman has experienced a G-spot orgasm. Even though the G-spot is about two inches inside the vagina, it can still be stimulated during oral sex.

Guys, here is the best way to find and stimulate her goddess spot. But before you begin, be sure your lover is well lubricated either naturally or from using some commercial lubricants like Wet or Astroglide. These are available at most pharmacies.

1. Begin by resting your thumb on her clitoris while inserting the middle finger of your prominent hand in a "come here" motion into her vagina, palm up.

2. Imagine there is a clock on the inside of your partner's vagina and you are stroking from 6 o'clock (at the bottom of her vaginal opening) to 12 o'clock (her G-spot). Use long strokes, creating an energetic circuit between your thumb and finger.

3. The goddess spot is about the size of a dime. It will feel different to the rest of the tissue inside the vagina. It will feel like it has ridges on it, much like corduroy material or the roof of your mouth.

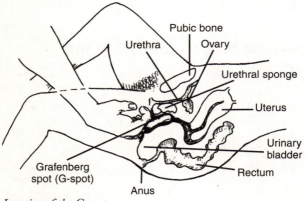

Location of the G-spot.

By stimulating her goddess spot and lavishing her clitoris with oral sex, you will help your lover achieve multiple orgasms—a clitoral orgasm and a goddess orgasm simultaneously—and guys, you will be a hero. So follow carefully:

1. Pull back the clitoral hood.

2. Lick the clitoris, alternating with short strokes directly on the clitoris and long strokes that start at the vaginal opening and end at the clitoris. Do this until she reaches a level 8 on her pleasure scale of 1 to 10. Remember, if she reaches a 10, you'll have to start all over again. Ask her to let you know when she's reached a level 8. Depending on your partner's personal sexual cycle, her response could take anywhere from 2 to 15 minutes. It has nothing to do with your performance.

3. Move your tongue away from the clitoris and stimulate the entire vaginal opening in circular tongue motions, from smaller to larger circles, licking every inch of her vaginal opening. Do this for a couple minutes only.

4. Go back to stimulating her clitoris with short and long strokes until she reaches a level 9 on her pleasure scale. Be sure she doesn't get carried away.

5. Now slip the middle finger of your prominent hand inside her vagina, palm up so you can find the goddess spot. Meanwhile, continue to lick her clitoris with only short strokes.

6. Once your finger is on top of her goddess spot, tap it toward the belly button, still maintaining oral stimulation on her clitoris.

7. Now you continue to tap her goddess spot and lick her clitoris rhythmically until she reaches her multiple orgasms.

This technique is one that will leave your lover exhausted, exhilarated, and extremely satisfied.

Vagina Talk

Stimulation of the clitoris (the primary sexual organ) and the breasts (the secondary sexual organ) at the same time can send women to orgasmic bliss. Do this in the 69 position with your penis in between her breasts instead of her mouth while you lick her clitoris.

The Least You Need to Know

- A man who can lick his lover from head to toe will be her hero in bed.

- Enthusiasm is still more important than technique, so let her know how much you want to go down on her.

- The female G-spot is not a myth. It comes from stimulating the urethral sponge; every woman has one.

- Women can have two separate kinds of orgasm, one external one from the clitoris, and one internal one from the G-spot.

Chapter 11

How to Rock His World

In This Chapter

- Make it visual
- How to deep-throat
- Sexually dominate him
- Find his H-spot

In this chapter, you'll learn advanced oral sex techniques that will make you a fellatio aficionado. You'll discover how to become a sex slave one minute and a dominatrix the next. Find out why men enjoy oral sex in the morning and how you can leave a lasting impression he'll never forget. You'll also be taught all about the male prostate, what his H-spot is, and how to stimulate it so he can experience multiple orgasms.

Most men will confess that erotic stimulation is about 70 percent visual and 30 percent physical. That should give you a clue as to what to do to rock his world. Bear in mind that men are not biologically programmed to be with one woman.

That means they have traditionally been able to get away with more than women in the way of boorish behavior. It's not fair, I know. But the bottom line is that you can gain the edge over a man's natural tendencies to play the field by keeping your sex life interesting.

Do anything you can do to be different, better, more creative, and adventurous, and don't be afraid to initiate sex, especially oral sex. If you want a monogamous man, you need to make it happen. Because men tend to become turned on visually, you can do a lot to bring a man to climax simply by using your body in imaginative ways.

Vamp It Up

The first step to vamping it up is to dress in sexy lingerie like low-cut bras, suspender hose, a G-string or transparent panties, thigh highs, and other assorted lingerie for your man's enjoyment. Don't forget the high-heeled stilettos. There's nothing more exciting for a man (no matter what age he is) than when he finds his date has stockings and a garter belt under her dress.

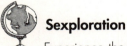

Sexploration

Experience the allure of dressing in stockings and titillating lingerie for yourself and discover how sexy you feel when you wear them.

Do a Striptease

The ultimate fantasy for a man is to watch his lover do a striptease for him. Your interpretation of the striptease depends solely on your mood and the image you wish to project—from artfully subtle to elegant, sexy, and chic, to lusty, wild, and X-rated. Your outfit is a provocative prelude to an ultra-hot coming attraction … you!

If you're still wrestling with shyness, rent some movies like *9 1/2 Weeks*, *True Lies*, *Striptease*, or *Showgirls*, and see how it's done. Once you get over the first-time jitters, you'll get as involved in the eroticism of the striptease as he will. Try it, you'll like it, and he'll love it!

Choose some music you can move to (Chapter 4 has some suggestions). Stand in front of your lover, maintaining eye contact with him. Rub your hands all over your fully clad body in slow motion and give him a seductive little smile. Then remove your dress and let it fall to the floor, step back, and let him admire your legs and body encased in the nylons and lingerie. Turn around so he can appreciate your rear framed by the garter belt and stockings. Bend over and wiggle your butt teasingly. Turn back toward him, and slink your way between his legs. Don't take off your shoes, even for oral sex, because they complete the outfit.

Cleavage Fornication

Hang your breasts over him and push them on his face, then down the rest of his body until you are kneeling on the floor with your breasts at the same level as his penis. This is guaranteed to get the proverbial rise out of him. Unzip his pants, if they are not already off, and place his penis between your breasts. Remove your bra or ask him to unsnap your bra for you as you continue to push your breasts together (this works no matter what size they are) and lift your breasts up and down with his penis tightly packed in the middle between them. This is called cleavage fornication, and men love it.

Become His Sex Slave

Make your man the center of your attention. Don't answer the phone while you're with him. If you're married with children, tell them Mom and Dad need to have their private play time, and leave them with someone who can take care of them while you take care of your man.

Let him know you want to be his sex slave for one hour (or more) and that you'll do anything he wants. I pretty much guarantee oral sex will be part of his pleasure plan for you. To add to this fantasy, you can refer to your lover as "Master."

Bodice Ripper

Instead of throwing out old undies, you can let your lover tear them off you and adoringly ravage you as part of your sex slave fantasy. If the material is too thick, cut it in strategic places so they tear off more easily. Pretend you are a centerfold model, and ask him to take some photos of you partially clad or completely nude. This little game can really get the juices flowing and rev up your sex life.

Deep-Throating

It will be in this sexual arena that most men will want to straddle their partner's face and penetrate her mouth with their penis for a deep-throat experience. If you are not adverse to this, lie down and throw your head back so you can open up your mouth and throat. Be sure you have plenty of saliva in your mouth, breath through your nose, and then try sliding his penis down your throat as far as it will go. In case you start to feel yourself gagging, have some lubricant ready to put on your hand so that it's wet, then take a hold of the base of his penis and use your hand as an extension of your mouth by rubbing it up and down to the same tempo as your mouth.

Another deep-throat technique is to twist your head in a circular motion, which requires more effort (and enthusiasm) for the girl to turn her head and neck while sucking the penis deeply.

Tea-Bagging

If deep-throating is not your bag, then you might consider tea-bagging. It's a term often used by gay men to describe dipping testicles into an eager and open mouth. As his sex slave, you can lie obediently beneath him and maneuver his testicles into your mouth. Start by running your tongue around each ball, licking it slowly, then change the rhythm to a faster, more intense licking until you are ready for the tea-bagging ceremony. Watch those teeth. Dip one at a time into your mouth, and remember his balls are delicate. Suck on it as if you were savoring the flavor of ripe plum, draining the juice out of it, without biting into it. If you think you can handle it, try to dip both of his balls into your mouth and lick with your tongue as you suck with your mouth. If your jaw can only stay wide open for a few moments, that will be enough to impress him so he'll always remember it and you.

Dominate Him

Ladies, if you've ever wanted a man to worship you and treat you like a goddess, you need to know how to unleash the tigress within you. I believe every woman has a dominatrix inside of her that wants to come out and play. Be bold and playful so you can become the confident and dominant woman you were created to be.

Dress up in your most erotic yet dominant outfit. Leather boots, a latex mini skirt, and black top are perfect. The outfit will help you get into character. Tell your man you want him totally naked before you. Make him bend over and spank his butt with your hairbrush, saying, "You've been a very bad boy so you have to be punished." Demand that he suck on your breasts, spread your labia, and lick your clit. Then tell him that if he doesn't do it well, he won't get a blow job. Be a bitch.

Once you have him in a place of submission, change your character. Go from aggressive to gentle. Hold him, kiss him, and tell him he's been a good boy. Take him to a comfortable bed or couch and have him lay down on his back.

Now tell him that the only way he's going to get a blow job is if he begs you for it. Just watch how aroused he gets with this kind of talk and role-playing. Most men enjoy some kind of female authority in the bedroom. When he says the word *please* you can circle your tongue around the head of his penis and gently tug on his testicles simultaneously. This is also a great way to get him to talk erotically to you. Encourage him to tell you what he likes and how he likes it. Alternatively, you can demand that he describe what you are doing to him in graphic detail. To heighten the sexual excitement, maintain eye contact with him.

- Lick his raphe (the seam that runs along the underside of the penis) with the flat of your tongue. Then press your tongue flat on his frenulum with his penis balancing on your tongue and hold it still for a few moments.

- Put your finger (palm up) inside his mouth while you slide his penis slowly into your mouth, pulling him in with your lips, moving back and forth. Suck him deeper with each forward motion.

- Change your rhythm from long, slow sucking to short, fast-milking action, making lots of slurping noises as you suck. Hold onto his hips or butt and pull him toward you as you increase the pace.

- Shake and wiggle his penis in your mouth as you create a vacuum suction with your lips.

- Pump his penis shaft with one (lubricated) hand while you concentrate on sucking the glans with short, intense motions.

The more he begs you, the more you should fellate him.

> **Oral Info** _____
>
> More mature men need greater pressure to get any specific sensation, while younger men mostly enjoy a lighter touch.

Morning Glory

It's a fact that most men wake up with an erection in the morning because they need to empty their bladder, but it's also a fact that men's sexual hormone levels are higher in the morning, which means they are ready for sexual activity. Even if you're not a morning person, give him a treat once in a while so he can go to work with a smile on his face and a swing in his walk.

When you first wake up, your mouth can feel as dry as a rock. If you drink something or suck on a candy, it will get the saliva flowing. There's nothing sexier than surprising your man with a morning blow job. Slide under the sheets and nestle in between his legs, where you can manipulate his penis with your hands and mouth. Start by caressing him with your fingertips by walking them up and down his shaft and around the tip. Then blow your warm breath up and down his penis, and around his testicles and anus area. Brush your hair against his penis and stroke your face with it. Hold the base as you taste him by licking around the coronal ridge. Flick your tongue back and forth over the frenulum. Then create a seal around his glans with your mouth as you let your tongue dance around it. As you do this, make light humming sounds to give him some extra vibration. This is a sure way to get him to return the favor and maybe even make you breakfast in bed.

His Inner H-Spot

The man's equivalent of a woman's G-spot is his *prostate gland*, which I like to call his "H-spot" for hero spot. Every man wants to feel like a hero in bed, so why not name a spot after him? I've been told by men that when they reach a climax through prostate gland stimulation combined with oral sex, it is an unforgettable, mind-blowing multi-orgasmic experience. But lacking a vagina, there is no direct route to it. You can reach it in two ways, however. One is by using your finger or dildo to reach into his anus—this is a little tricky, so be sure he is willing to tell you when it is "feeling good." This point is about one to two inches inside the anus.

Penis Talk

The **prostate gland** is about the size of a walnut. It surrounds the urethra and is at the neck of the bladder. This gland produces the majority of the ejaculatory fluid expelled in semen.

Before you start, be sure to lubricate your finger and then gently ease it into him, keeping in mind that just an inch or so of penetration will get you to his H-spot. If you use your finger to reach inside him, buy some latex finger cots at the drugstore, which are ideal for this purpose. They can be easily lubricated and just as easily discarded after use to prevent the potential spread of bacteria from the anal area.

The best positions for finding his H-spot are either for him to lie on his back with a pillow under his butt and knees raised so you can lie between his thighs and rest your head on one of them, or he can get down on all fours so you can stimulate him from behind. Here are step-by-step instructions on how to find his H-spot and give him oral sex in unison:

1. Insert your finger palm up (as in discovering the G-spot) in a "come here" motion.

2. Once your finger is inside the anus, feel around for a raised nub, which is the prostate gland. Maintain good communication with your partner, and ask him to let you know how it feels. Ask him to use the pleasure scale from Chapter 7 on orgasms.

3. Once you've found his H-spot, start tapping it toward the navel in quick succession.

4. Meanwhile, lick his perineum with long, lapping strokes as if you were licking on an ice-cream cone.

Alternatively, you can suck on his testicles, one at a time or both together, while stimulating his H-spot.

Another technique is to do the good old fashioned up-and-down sucking of his penis while stimulating his H-spot.

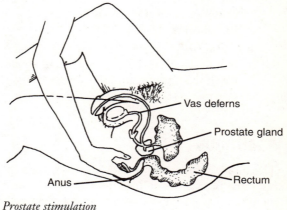

Prostate stimulation

His Outer H-Spot

You can also stimulate his H-spot by rubbing on his perineum, just below his testicles. Remember that men aren't as sensitive to pressure as women, so there's no need to be overly gentle when massaging this area (unless he asks you to lighten up).

1. Start your anal exploration by lightly circling the outside of his anus with your fingers or tongue. You can also try using a small vibrator like the Pocket Rocket.

2. Push your three middle fingers (preferably lubricated), onto the external H-spot, kneading the area as if were pizza dough.

Press in and out, circle one way, then the other, and observe his body language.

3. In the meantime, use your mouth to stimulate his penis by sucking him from the base to the glans in slow motion. Take your time to arouse him to a fever pitch.

4. As his breathing increases, so should your tempo. Don't forget not to change your rhythm before he climaxes unless he asks you to.

Analingus

The most exciting position for a man to receive oral-anal pleasure is on his knees bending over. I've mentioned cleanliness and the risks of giving oral sex around the anus in several chapters. I cannot reiterate the warning enough that analingus can result in contagious STDs; however, it can also be a highly erotic experience. You can use some plastic wrap over the anus or (if you are in a healthy monogamous relationship) take a shower or a bath with your lover so you both feel, look, and taste squeaky clean. Here's what you need to do:

1. Hold your lover's butt and spread his cheeks slightly apart to expose more of his anus. Because it's a power-packed little bud of erogenous sensitivity, start to lick around the anus with the tip of your tongue clockwise and counterclockwise.

2. Lick up and down over it with the flat of your tongue and side to side over it with the side of your tongue.

3. If your lover's response is positive, and the experience is a turn-on for you, go ahead and penetrate the tip of your tongue inside the anus and push it in and out with quick darting motions.

You can replace your tongue with your finger at any time.

Sexploration

Lots of men love anal play once they're introduced to it by a loving woman. However, some ladies are a bit shy in doing this. My advice is: Get over it. Attitudes like this are why guys sometimes cheat on "nice girls."

The Least You Need to Know

- Men love to be seduced visually, so put on your sexiest lingerie and high heels, and do a striptease if you can.
- Deep-throating is a common sexual fantasy for most men because they love to watch their penis disappear into a woman's mouth and go down her throat as far as it can.
- Men's sexual hormone levels are higher in the morning, so give him an oral treat in bed or in the shower before he goes to work.
- The prostate gland (equivalent to the female G-spot) can be located one to two inches through the anus, but use plenty of lubrication so you don't hurt him.

Chapter 12

Sexercise

In This Chapter

- Penis elongation and vagina aerobics
- Tongue stretches
- Exercises to sustain an erection
- Masturbation exercises for him and her

In the chapter, you'll learn how to keep your genitals in tip-top condition. We all know that regular exercise helps keep our body in good shape. But not everyone knows the importance of exercising their sexual organs. In this chapter, you'll learn how to strengthen the penis, vagina, and surrounding muscles so they can operate at their full potential. Tongue stretches will prepare you for the Oral Olympics. Sexercise for couples to do together are guaranteed to improve intimacy as well as physical endurance. Mandatory masturbation exercises are all part of the program. Whether you choose to do these sexercises solo or with your partner, the benefits will result in better sexual performance, bigger orgasms, and more sexual confidence.

The Penis Elongation Workout

How many of you take the time to stretch every day? It's good for you to extend your back and your limbs. It can prevent you from having bad posture; it can relieve pain in your muscles and strengthen your physique. The same is true when you stretch the penis. There is extra skin at the base of the penis just behind the scrotum that is ready, willing, and waiting to be stretched.

Penis enlargement is not a myth. Elongation exercises have been performed in parts of Asia and Africa for centuries. Stretching the penis is the most practical and safest way to increase the length with lasting results.

If the penis is stretched regularly, the tissue will elongate and can add permanent length to it, so if length is what you're after, here's an exercise that can help you get it naturally:

1. Lie on your back, legs spread, or sit on the edge of a chair. It's also a good idea to do this in front of a mirror.

2. The penis should be flaccid and, if uncircumcised, the foreskin should be pulled back before starting.

3. Holding the glans, stretch the penis upward (toward the navel), and hold for a count of 10.

4. Repeat this stretch and then hold in the downward position (toward the feet), and hold for another count of 10.

5. Then to the left and to the right, both times for a count of 10.

This exercise should be done two times a day for five minutes.

Scrotum Sexercise

The two glands that are protected by the scrotum hang beneath the penis and manufacture precious sperm, testosterone, and other male hormones. It's important to examine your reproductive organs regularly and to exercise the testes along with the penis.

Lift the scrotum upward and hold against your body for 10 seconds. When done properly, your penis should press against your stomach. Then release, relax, and repeat. Your goal is to work up to six minutes of repetitions twice a day.

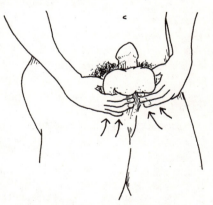

Lift your scrotum upward, and hold it against your body.

Vagina Aerobics

For women who have trouble achieving an orgasm, there may be an answer—doing a series of simple exercises I like to call Vagina Aerobics. These exercises were originally developed by Dr. Arnold Kegel to strengthen bladder control for women suffering from incontinence (when urine continues to drip after emptying the bladder). Today, Kegel exercises are highly recommended for pregnant women so they strengthen the pelvic floor muscles that support the bowel, bladder, and womb to make it easier to deliver. But it's also important to note that Kegels are not only for expecting mothers; these exercises can help keep the vagina tight and elastic so love-making is more enjoyable for both partners.

If you are one of the 35 to 75 percent of all women who have difficulty in climaxing during intercourse, you should know that your ability to reach an orgasm correlates with the tightening of your *pubococcygeus (PC) muscle*. Because it is the master muscle of the pelvis, strong PC muscles result in strong orgasms and weak PC muscles don't.

Vagina Talk

The **pubococcygeus (PC) muscles** can be as thin as a pinky finger or as thick as three fingers. You want it to be thick and strong so it can help keep the vagina toned and tight. When the PC muscles are weak, the pelvic organs it supports are inclined to sag, which can lead to urinary incontinence (uncontrollable bladder leakage) and sexual problems.

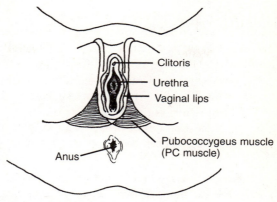

Female PC Muscles.

First you need to identify your PC muscles. If you don't know where they are, the next time you go to the bathroom to urinate, do the following exercise. Sit on the toilet and start to urinate, then stop and start the flow of urine as many times as you can. This is the only muscle that can accomplish this. Don't try to use your thighs, abdomen, or buttocks. A good self-check is to insert one finger into the vagina and feel the muscles contracting as you squeeze. Once you have identified the PC muscles, you no longer need to urinate to exercise it. You can do these exercises anywhere: while driving, eating, talking on the phone, or waiting in line, not to mention while making love! Here are your vagina aerobics. Do them daily and you'll feel orgasmic results like never before.

- Squeeze and hold the PC muscles for 3 seconds, relax, and repeat for 20 repetitions 2 times a day.

- Tighten and relax your PC muscles 10 times in rapid succession. Repeat this three times, two times a day.

- Lie down on the floor for this exercise and take a deep breath. Then pull up your pelvis by visualizing that you are sucking water into your vagina. Hold for three seconds, then push out or bear down as if you are trying to push the water out of your vagina.

All these exercises should be done regularly. However, the PC muscles are like any other muscles, and if you are too vigorous at first, they can become sore. Always listen to your body and do fewer repetitions if you ache too much. Within a couple months, you should feel a greater sensation during intercourse.

Tickle the Kitty

Female masturbation is a natural, healthy sexual activity that more than 15 percent of women do not pursue because they don't know what to do or they feel guilty and shameful about it. Not only is masturbation good for you physically, but psychologically it can boost your self-esteem, make you more sexually confident, and help you communicate your sexual needs to your partner.

In preparation for masturbation, you can do exercises that I like to call *tickle the kitty*. It's a good idea to conjure up an erotic fantasy. Lie down, close your eyes, and picture yourself in a sexual act you've always wanted to experience. You can imagine that you are being watched, you are being restrained, or even making-love with a celebrity. A fantasy is a safe place, and there's no need to feel guilty about it.

Start by licking your fingers to make them wet. Touch your body all over and spread your legs as your fingers make their way down to your vulva. Stimulate your clitoris with a combination of strokes, and explore what motions feel best for you. Many women can reach an orgasm from stimulating the clitoris in circular rubbing motions. Others prefer stroking the sides of the clitoris. It's up to you to find out what turns you on the most.

Sexploration

Observing each other giving self-pleasure is educational, highly erotic, and it's a safe sex activity. I encourage couples to engage in mutual masturbation because it's a great way to find out where your partner likes to be touched and how he or she enjoys being stimulated. Mutual masturbation will be a lot easier to do if you masturbate on your own first.

If you need a little extra help, you can use a vibrator like the Pocket Rocket by Doc Johnson, a handy little vibrator designed specifically for clitoral stimulation, or a dildo for full vaginal or anal penetration. There is no right or wrong way to masturbate, but I do recommend variety. Masturbate in different positions and on different objects like a pillow, a rolled up sock, even the tumble dryer on spin cycle. Use a different hand or enjoy the stimulation of a water faucet or shower massager on your genitals. Surrender yourself to the experience of orgasmic pleasure. Tickle the kitty at least three times a week.

Tongue Territory

Our tongue is a multifunctional organ with countless muscles that can lick, suck, slurp, wet, roll, twist, and tease our lover. Without our tongue, we couldn't talk, chew, swallow, or sing. Just try eating an ice-cream cone without using your tongue and you'll find out how difficult a task it is.

> **Oral Info**
>
> The tongue has a thin mucous membrane called the frenulum, just like the underside of the penis. It's located in the middle on the undersurface of the tongue. If you open your mouth and lift your tongue, you'll see the lingual frenulum.

Tongue Stretches

Because the tongue is so flexible with all its muscles, it's important to maintain its agility, especially if you want to be a master or mistress at giving oral sex. Follow these exercises, and do them once daily or just before an oral sex adventure:

- Extend your tongue between your lips as far as you can. Hold it steady and straight for 10 seconds. Relax and repeat three times. You may not want to do this in public.

- Retract your tongue, lifting the back of it to the roof of your mouth. Hold for five seonds. Relax and repeat three times.

- Stretch out your tongue, move it to the right as far as you can. Hold it for five seconds. Relax and repeat two times.

- Stretch out your tongue, move it to the left as far as you can. Hold it for five seconds. Relax and repeat two times.

- Move your tongue to the far left and then far right as fast as you can. Repeat 20 times.

- Stretch your tongue out and up to the tip of your nose. Hold for three seconds. Relax and repeat two times.

- Stretch your tongue out and down toward your chin. Hold for three seconds. Relax and repeat two times.

These tongue exercises may seem funny, but don't underestimate the power of your tongue when it comes to oral sex.

Tongue Piercing

Tongue piercing is growing in popularity, but think about the risks before you have a needle penetrate your tongue. There have been reports of pain, impaired speech, loss of taste and tongue mobility, and infections after tongue piercing, not to mention fractured teeth from metal tongue jewelry. Just because famous people like Janet Jackson and Billy Idol have their tongues pierced, doesn't mean it's right for you. Don't get me wrong, I know how truly erotic it can be for the piercee and his or her partner. Simply running the barbell stud along the shaft of his penis or rolling the little metal stud around the clitoris can drive your lover wild. But the bottom line is that you have mutilated your tongue and you can also drive your lover wild with other oral sex techniques found in this book.

Love Muscle Exercises for Men

The love muscle is clinically known as the *pubococcygeus muscles*, but we'll call it PC for short. It's the same muscle the ladies used for their Vagina Aerobics. These muscles are the support muscles for the genitals in both men and women. There is a definite correlation between good tone in the PC muscles and orgasmic intensity and control. A quick way to identify the PC muscles is to urinate, then stop the flow of urine by squeezing your PC muscles, without using your thighs, abdomen, or sphincter (muscular ring at the entrance of the anus) muscles, then urinate again. After a few repetitions, most people are able to tighten these muscles without the involvement of urination.

The benefits of having strong PC muscles increase blood flow to the genitals, help tone the prostate gland, and can result in separating orgasm from ejaculation. Now you know why I refer to them as love muscles.

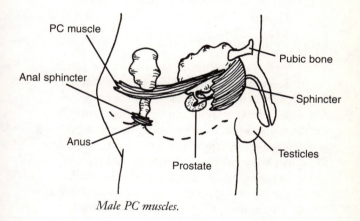

Penis Talk

The **pubococcygeus (PC) muscle** is part of the sling of muscles expanding from the pubic bone to the tailbone. This is like any other muscle in the body that needs to be strengthened. A strong, healthy PC will give you a strong, healthy erection that will last as long as you want it to.

PC muscle

Pubic bone

Anal sphincter

Sphincter

Anus

Testicles

Prostate

Male PC muscles.

Solo Penis Exercises

If you do the following exercises regularly, you'll be able to make love for as long as you want without ejaculating, and here's the icing on the cake—you'll still be able to experience a full-body orgasm!

- Lie down on your back or sit in a chair and get comfortable. Using plenty of lubrication, begin stroking your penis and experiencing your arousal level rise. Your arousal level will vary from level (1), which is barely aroused, to level (10), which is when you would typically orgasm and ejaculate. It's important for you to recognize each level of arousal. Practice squeezing your PC muscles, stopping and starting at each level of your arousal from 1 to 10. This is like one big tease after another. It's also a great excuse for masturbation.

- Put your fingers on each side of the shaft so you can feel the PC muscles contracting. Then squeeze the PC muscles for 20 repetitions. Do this two times a day.

- For the next exercise, you'll need an erection. Place a light scarf, handkerchief, or towel over the base of your erect penis (Exercise 1) and use your PC muscles to lift it up and down, like a weight, for 20 repetitions. (You may want to start with a tissue and work your way up to a dry towel, then a wet towel.) After completing the first set of lifts, move the towel to the head of the penis (Exercise 2), and raise it up and down for 20 more repetitions. Do these two times a day.

- Once you've successfully identified your PC muscles, you can practice squeezing them during the day while you're driving, sitting in your office, waiting in line at the grocery store, or just talking on the phone. You won't need an erection, and nobody will know what you're doing. Just tighten your PC muscles and hold for a count of three, then relax. Do 20 reps a day, 2 times a day. Alternate by doing slow squeezes then rapid squeezes.

For rapid squeezes, tighten and relax your PC muscles as quickly as you can, and do as many as you can in 60 seconds 2 times a day.

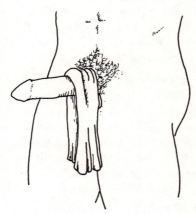

Penis towel exercise 1.

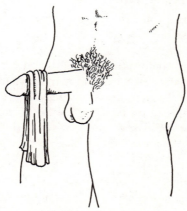

Penis towel exercise 2.

Charm the Snake

Who would have thought masturbation would be a recommended exercise? I'm here to tell you that regular masturbation is good for your health, whether you are in a relationship or not. I like to call this exercise *charming the snake* because the idea is to make your penis stand up for as long as you can.

Time how long it takes you to reach your orgasm by watching a clock or counting the strokes. For best results, do both. Then try to extend it each time you masturbate. If on average you reach your climax in 50 strokes and in 2 minutes, then strive for 60 strokes and 2 minutes and 30 seconds the next time you charm the snake. Give yourself a realistic goal you can strive for. Most men can double the strokes and the time within one month.

Am I Coming or Going?

The exercises you already read about will help men who suffer from premature ejaculation. More than 50 percent of all men experience some kind of erection problem before the age of 40. Did you know that one of the reasons a man may suffer from premature ejaculation is because when he was a young boy he probably masturbated too fast for fear of getting caught? When adulthood is reached, those old habits are still there, and it's hard (excuse the pun) to give up old habits.

Another tried-and-true exercise to help prevent premature ejaculation is called the squeeze technique. You can grasp the glans (head of the penis) with two fingers underneath and the thumb on top or squeeze the base of the penis. Experiment with both the head and the base to see which one works best for you. This should be done for approximately five seconds every time you feel the urge to ejaculate.

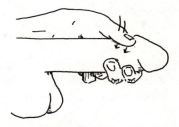

Squeeze the head of the penis.

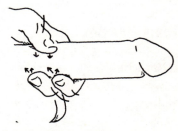

Squeeze the base of the penis.

Similarly, there is a stop-start technique, which is exactly that. Stimulate yourself—stop—stimulate—stop—stimulate—stop. The stops should last for five seconds.

Retarded or delayed ejaculation (the same problem) is the opposite of premature ejaculation. It is when someone has difficulty ejaculating. Inhibitions, lack of stimulation, religious repression, fear of impregnation, alcohol, or other drugs and medications often cause retarded or delayed ejaculation. Know-ing your penis and exercising it regularly can prevent erectile problems.

Sexploration

Did you know that for a healthy penis you should have three erections and two orgasms per week to ensure it's getting the oxygen it needs? For a healthy vagina, you should have at least two orgasms a week. Eat veg-etables, drink plenty of water, and reduce your fat intake. And everyone should exer-cise their PC muscles regularly!

Partner Penis Exercises

Turn these penis exercises into an adult game, and share the rules with your lover so she can play along with you.

Partner Penis Exercise 1: This exercise begins with the man lying on his back. Ask your partner to begin caressing your penis gently and slowly with her hands. Do a series of low-level peaks from level 1 to level 6 just the way you did with your solo exercises. Give your partner lots of feedback so she knows when to back off and when to intensify her caresses.

Partner Penis Exercise 2: Now do Exercise 1 again, except ask your partner to stimulate your penis with her mouth this time. Do a series of peaks from 1 to 7, and try to maintain control by communicating with your partner when she should stop and when she should intensify her licking and sucking. Once you have completed these peaks without ejaculating, switch positions. She'll think this is fun, too.

Partner Penis Exercise 3: This time get into the traditional 69 position. Do a series of peaks while giving and receiving oral sex simultaneously. Start with some slow licking, and ask your partner to do the same. Do a series of peaks from 1 to 8 as you speed up your oral practice. Don't forget, the higher the peak, the harder you have to squeeze your PC muscles. If you feel yourself getting carried away, stop moving, slow down your breathing, and, if necessary, focus only on giving your lover oral sex for a while. This will take your focus off your erection, but it will not deplete completely. Then return to having mutual oral sex until your partner has her orgasm and you peak up to a level 9 on your arousal scale. This is almost to your point of no return. Now squeeze your PC muscles as hard as you can, take deep breaths, open your eyes, focus all your attention on your genitals, and try to mentally prevent the semen from moving from your testicles to the base of your penis. Ask your lover to stop giving your oral sex because any extra motion right now could cause you to ejaculate before you want to. If you stopped in time, you should feel an orgasmic ripple from your head to your toes. You will have experienced an orgasm without ejaculation. Congratulations!

Once you master this technique, you can prolong your orgasm for as long as you like and you can control when you have an orgasm and when you ejaculate. This technique takes lots of practice and self-control. My advice: "If at first you don't succeed, try, try again."

The first few times you try these exercises, you may feel any number of unfamiliar sensations, such as a partial orgasm or even a *skipped* orgasm (having no orgasm at all). Be patient, because your body is learning new things and these sensations are quite normal.

The Least You Need to Know

- Penis elongation exercises can extend the penis when done on a regular basis.

- Women who have difficulty reaching an orgasm should do Kegel exercises every day because there is a connection between tightening the PC muscle and reaching an orgasm.

- Doing tongue stretches before oral sex will help maintain its agility and staying power when giving oral sex.

- Exercising the PC muscles for men increases blood flow to the genitals, tones the prostate gland, and can result in separating orgasm from ejaculation.

- Use the "squeeze technique" (squeezing the base or head of the penis) to prevent premature ejaculation.

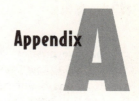

Glossary

amrita   female ejaculation fluid.

anal sex   Sexual contact and/or penetration with the anus.

aphrodisiac   A substance that is alleged to stimulate or increase sexual desire.

areola   Pigmented area that surrounds the nipple on the breasts.

butt plug   Sex toy for the anus.

circumcision   The surgical removal of foreskin of the penis.

clap   Gonorrhea.

cleavage fornication   Stimulation of the penis in between the breasts.

climaxing   The point at which orgasm occurs.

clitoral stimulation   To touch the clitoris sexually.

clitoris   A small organ located at the point where the labia minora connect. It plays a vital role in a woman's sexual arousal.

come   To experience orgasm; semen; ejaculation.

consensual sex   Sex as a mutual agreement between two people.

contraception   Birth control.

coronal ridge   The ridge around the head of the penis.

corpus cavernosum   Fills up with blood when stimulated and allows for erection to take place.

corpus spongiosum   A cavity located in the penis that fills with blood during the ejaculatory process.

crura   Part of the clitoris that is made up of two small "wings."

cunniligus   Oral stimulation of a woman's vulva, clitoris, and/or vagina.

deep-throat   A form of oral sex in which the penis is voluntarily taken deeply into the recipient's throat.

delayed ejaculation   Sufferers of delayed or retarded ejaculation find it difficult to ejaculate.

dental dams   Thin squares of latex usually used by dentists but are also used for safer sex practices, especially on women for oral sex.

depilatory cream   Hair removing cream.

dildo   An artificial substitute for an erect penis, made of silicone, rubber, or latex, designed for vaginal or anal insertion for sexual pleasure.

doggie style   A sexual position with man penetrating woman from the rear.

douche   A vaginal rinse.

ejaculation   The expulsion of semen from the penis.

endorphins   A group of peptide hormones found mainly in the brain. Endorphins can reduce the sensation of pain and affect emotions.

epididymis   Coiled tubes located on the side of the testicles that carry new sperm.

erection   Enlargement of the penis when blood flowing to the area causes it to become engorged.

erogenous zones   Areas of the body and skin that respond to sexual stimulation.

fallopian tubes   Two tubes located in the female reproductive system, that lead to the uterus.

fellatio   Oral sexual stimulation of the penis.

female condom   A disposable tube of polyurethane and plastic rings that is inserted into the vagina over the cervix.

female prostatic fluid   Female ejaculation.

fetish   Something such as a material object (shoes) or a nonsexual part of the body (feet) that arouses sexual desire and may become necessary for sexual gratification.

foreplay   Sexual stimulation that happens before intercourse.

foreskin   A fold of thin skin that hangs over the glans of the penis in uncircumcised men.

frenulum   The part of penis linking the foreskin to the penis, located in the ridge under the glans of the penis.

gag reflex   The biological reflex that causes someone to feel like they are choking when the back of their throat is stimulated.

genitals   The reproductive organs.

glans   The head of the penis.

goddess spot   *See* G-spot.

G-spot   First identified by Dr. Ernst Grafenburg and located on the front of the inner upper wall of the vagina, which can result in orgasm when stimulated.

hymen   A membrane at the entrance to the woman's vagina.

hypoallergenic   Minimizes the likelihood of causing an allergic response.

impotence   A man's inability to achieve or maintain an erection of sufficient firmness for penetration during intercourse.

intercourse   The act of sexual procreation between a man and a woman. Also known as copulation.

Kegel exercises Repeated contractions and release of the pubococcygeus (PC) muscles to strengthen them and increase sexual sensitivity; developed by Dr. Arnold Kegel.

labia majora The outer vaginal lips.

labia minora The inner vaginal lips.

lubricants Solutions that lessen or prevent friction.

masturbation Self-stimulation of one's own genitals for sexual pleasure.

menstruation The discharge of blood and tissue from the lining of the uterus through the vagina for about three to seven days each month.

missionary position A sexual position in which the man is on top of the woman.

monogamy A sexually exclusive relationship, usually as part of a committed relationship.

mons The soft area above the vagina that is covered with pubic hair.

mons veneris The pubic hair area.

multiple orgasms More than one orgasm at a time or in close succession of each other.

mutual masturbation Sexual contact in which people manually stimulate each other's genitals at the same time.

nipple The tips of the breasts in men and women.

Nonoxynol-9 spermicide A spermicide widely used in contraceptive creams, foams, and lubricants.

oral copulation Sexual stimulation of the male or female genitals using the mouth.

orgasm Sexual climax, marked by blood flow to the genitals, involuntary rhythmic contraction of the pelvic muscles and erotic pleasure.

ovaries   Two glands in the female reproductive system that produce eggs during the monthly cycle and hormones that are involved in sexual response development of secondary sex characteristics.

pearl necklace   A deposit of semen around the neck.

pelvic floor   A series of muscles that form a sling across the opening of the pelvis.

penetration   The act of piercing or penetrating something, especially a vagina with a penis or a tongue.

penis   Male reproductive and sex organ.

perineum   The area of skin between the genitals and the anus in both men and women.

periurethral sponge   *See* G-spot.

plateau   A stage of the sexual response cycle in which the excitement maintains a high level prior to climaxing to the orgasm stage.

pornography   Written, spoken, or visual material that stimulates sexual feelings.

pre-come   *See* pre-ejaculatory fluid.

pre-ejaculatory fluid   Fluid secreted by the man's Cowper's glands and discharged from his penis during arousal, prior to ejaculation.

premature ejaculation   Ejaculation before the man wants it to occur.

prepuce   Protective tissue that covers the clitoris.

prostaglandin-E   Hormone that helps men to maintain erection.

prostate exam   Exam that a doctor performs on a man by inserting a gloved lubricated finger into the man's rectum to feel his prostate and detect abnormalities.

prostate gland   A walnut-size gland located below the bladder in a man. It produces that majority of the fluid that combines with sperm and other secretions to make up semen.

prostatectomy   Surgical removal of excess prostate tissue, or in a radical prostatectomy, the removal of the prostate gland.

pubococcygeus (PC) muscles   Pelvic muscles that extend from the pubic bone in the front, around both sides of the sex organs, and back to the tailbone. Control over the PC muscles can enhance sexual response in women and men.

raphe   The seam that runs along the underside of the penis.

rear entry   The sexual position in which the man enters the woman's vagina from behind. Also called "doggie style."

resolution   The final stage of the sexual response cycle, which occurs after orgasm. During this stage, the body returns to the stage it was in prior to excitement.

retarded ejaculation   Sufferers of retarded ejaculation find it difficult to ejaculate. Also known as delayed ejaculation.

rimming   Oral-anal sexual contact.

role-playing   Acting out different roles, often for variety in sexual play.

sadomasochism (S/M or S&M)   A broad term applied to a number of activities such as physical restraining and erotic pain typically involving exchange of power or pain between consenting partners.

saliva   Secretion produced by salivary gland in the mouth.

scrotum   The pouch of skin that hangs below the penis and contains the testes.

semen   Fluid containing sperm that is expelled from the penis during ejaculation. Also called "ejaculate."

seminal vesicles   Two pouches in the male reproductive system, which secrete about 30 percent of the liquid portion of semen.

seminiferous tubes   Tightly coiled tubes located inside each of the testes.

sexual consent   Mutual agreement to have sex.

sexual fantasy   Image of sexual scenario that one creates with one's imagination.

sexual inhibitions   Sexual blocks or suppression.

sexuality   All aspects of one's personality and behaviors that are affected by being male or female.

shaft   Part of penis that extends from the head to beneath the hood.

shrimping   The act of sucking on toes.

sixty-niner   Simultaneous oral sex.

sodomy   Anal or oral penetration.

sperm   The male reproductive cell that is contained in semen, released during ejaculation, and may be united with a woman's egg to cause fertilization and to create life.

spermicide   Products that kill sperm to prevent pregnancy.

sphincter   The muscular ring at the entrance of the anus.

STD   Abbreviation for sexually transmitted disease that can be transmitted through sexual contact.

sterilization   Medical operations performed on men and women to prevent the possibility of reproduction.

taint   Slang term for the perineum.

tea-bagging   Dipping his testicles into your mouth.

testicles (testes)   Two small, oval glands in the scrotum that produce sperm and male hormones.

TriGasm   An orgasm that results from stimulation of three points of pleasure simultaneously.

unilateral copulation   When only one person gives oral sex to another without reciprocation.

unprotected sex   Sex without contraception or protection from STDs.

urethra   The canal that carries urine from the bladder.

uterus   An internal organ of the female reproductive system; also known as the womb.

vagina   The muscular passageway that leads from the uterus to the vulva. The area that receives the penis during sexual intercourse.

vagina aerobics   Kegel exercises to improve vaginal elasticity.

vaginal discharge   Unnatural secretions of the vagina that pertain to some kind of infection.

vas deferens   Two narrow tubes that convey sperm to the point where it can mix with the other constituents that make up semen.

vasectomy   A surgical method of permanent birth control (sterilization) that involves cutting and tying the vas deferens so a man does not ejaculate sperm yet he still ejaculates semen.

vestibule glands   Any of the glands that open into the vestibule of the vagina.

vibrator   An electric or battery-operated vibrating device that is often intended for stimulation of the genitals but can be used to massage other parts of the body.

virgin   One who has not had sexual intercourse.

vulva   Refers to all the external female sexual parts including the mons veneris, the labia majora and minora, the clitoris, the Bartholin's glands, the urethral opening, and vaginal openings.

yeast infection   An infection of the mucous membranes caused by the fungus *Candida albicans* inside the vagina.

Further Reading and Resources

I believe that even the best lovers can still learn and improve their techniques. The pages that follow list some of the best videos, sex education organizations, and online mail-order sites to make it easy for you to find out more information on your own.

The Best Videos on Oral Sex

The advantage of watching a video on oral sex is that you can observe someone giving it and getting it. You'll be able to emulate exactly what they are doing. Some of the following videos are extremely graphic, so not only will you learn the art of oral sex, but you'll probably get aroused at the same time. And, that's not a bad combination.

Hartley, Nina. Nina Hartley's Guide to Better Fellatio. California: Adam & Eve Productions 1994. Hall of Fame porn star Nina Hartley teaches and personally demonstrates various fellatio techniques. She gives her own personal insights on arousing your partner, and shares her years of sexual experience.

Hartley, Nina. Nina Hartley's Guide to Better Cunnilingus. California: Adam & Eve Productions 1994.
Celebrating a decade of erotic performing, Nina Hartley wrote and directed this video for everyone interested in expanding their sexual horizon and pleasing their mate orally.

Sinclair Intimacy Institute. Better Oral Sex Techniques. Sinclair Intimacy Institute, 1997.
The Sinclair Institute has released a guide to cunnilingus and fellatio as part of their series on how-to tapes. It features sex experts Dr. Marty Klein and Dr. Diana Wiley who introduce basic techniques that can help couples master cunnilingus and fellatio. Couples demonstrate oral sex on each other, and viewers can discover new ways to enjoy oral delights.

Dodson, Betty. Betty Dodson's Celebrating Orgasm. Pacific Media Entertainment, 2000.
This video is a great teaching tool for women and those who love them. Betty Dodson personally guides women on how to orgasm and how to get in touch with themselves sexually. The result is "Seven Techniques for Achieving Orgasmic Ecstasy, the foundation of Celebrating Orgasm."

Perry, Dr. Michael. Sexual Secrets a Sex Surrogate's Guide to Great Lovemaking. BCI Eclipse Company, 1994.
Sex therapist Dr. Michael Perry has produced a series of sex educational videos titled *The Intimacy Guide for Couples*. In this video, you'll see a sex surrogate teach some hot techniques on giving and getting oral sex. Other lessons include sex talk, sexual positions, and intercourse.

Sex Education and Therapy

Whether you're interested in finding out the answer to a pressing sex question, looking for a sex therapist in your neighborhood, or interested in becoming a sexologist yourself, the list of sex education resources here will lead you in the right direction.

The Institute for Advanced Study of Human Sexuality

This graduate school is one of the few in the world approved to train clinical sexologists. They also have an impressive sex museum where you can trace the history of sex. For more information on their degrees, you can call 415-928-1133 or go to their website at www.iashs.edu.

Sexuality Information and Education Council of the United States (SIECUS)

SIECUS is a national nonprofit organization that affirms that sexuality is a natural and healthy part of living. It develops, collects, and circulates information on sex education and advocates the right of individuals to make responsible sexual choices. For more information call 212-819-9770 or visit www.siecus.org.

The American Association of Sex Educators, Counselors, and Therapists (AASECT)

AASECT is a nonprofit, interdisciplinary professional organization. If you are looking for a sex educator, sexologist, sex counselor, or sex therapist, AASECT can help you find one they have certified in your area. Members of AASECT share an interest in promoting understanding of human sexuality and healthy sexual behavior. Call 804-644-3288, or go to www.aasect.org.

American Association of Marriage and Family Therapists (AAMFT)

The AAMFT Directory will assist you in locating a marriage and family therapist in your area. The listed therapists are clinical members of the American Association for Marriage and Family Therapy. The directory provides information on the therapist's office locations and availability, practice description, education, professional licenses, health plan participation, achievements and awards, and languages spoken. Call 202-452-0109, or visit www.aamft.org.

Mail-Order and Online Stores

Lots of people feel uncomfortable going to a sex shop, especially if they live in a small town where everyone knows each other. Now there's a better way to purchase your sex toys and sensual lingerie. It's anonymous, and it's easy.

Adam and Eve Catalog

This is one of the largest catalogs in the adult industry. You'll find the latest sex toys, sex education videos, adult DVDs, safer sex supplies, and lingerie. Call 1-800-274-0333 or go to their website at www.adameve.com.

Good Vibrations

This is a retail store located in San Francisco that has a catalog and a website where you can find information on sexual health, pleasure, and current events. You can also purchase sex toys, sex education, erotic and how-to books, and adult videos. Call 1-800-289-8423, or visit www.goodvibes.com.

Xandria Collection

For more than 30 years, the Xandria Collection has been one of America's top resources for sex toys, lingerie, and sex education. On their website, you can ask questions, learn about the history of sex, read jokes, or buy some sexy ecards. Call 1-800-242-2823 or go to www.xandria.com.

Toys in Babeland

This is a sex toy store run by women whose mission is to promote and celebrate sexual vitality by providing an honest, open, and fun environment. They not only offer the latest sex gadgets, but lingerie, lotions, and safer sex supplies, and you can even join one of their workshops. Call 1-800-658-9119, or check them out at www.toysinbabeland.com.

Index

W–X–Y–Z